Zoonoses, Public Health and the Exotic Animal Practitioner

Guest Editor

MARCY J. SOUZA, DVM, MPH, Dipl. ABVP–Avian, Dipl. ACVPM

VETERINARY CLINICS OF NORTH AMERICA: EXOTIC ANIMAL PRACTICE

www.vetexotic.theclinics.com

Consulting Editor
AGNES E. RUPLEY, DVM, Dipl. ABVP–Avian

September 2011 • Volume 14 • Number 3

SAUNDERS an imprint of ELSEVIER, Inc.

W.B. SAUNDERS COMPANY
A Division of Elsevier Inc.

1600 John F. Kennedy Boulevard • Suite 1800 • Philadelphia, Pennsylvania 19103-2899

http://www.vetexotic.theclinics.com

VETERINARY CLINICS OF NORTH AMERICA: EXOTIC ANIMAL PRACTICE Volume 14, Number 3
September 2011 ISSN 1094-9194, ISBN-13: 978-1-4557-1040-9

Editor: John Vassallo; j.vassallo@elsevier.com
Developmental Editor: Teia Stone

Veterinary Clinics of North America: Exotic Animal Practice (ISSN 1094-9194) is published in January, May, and September by Elsevier, Inc., 360 Park Avenue South, New York, NY 10010-1710. Subscription prices are $212.00 per year for US individuals, $345.00 per year for US institutions, $108.00 per year for US students and residents, $253.00 per year for Canadian individuals, $407.00 per year for Canadian institutions, $285.00 per year for international individuals, $407.00 per year for international institutions and $139.00 per year for Canadian and foreign students/ residents. To receive student/resident rate, orders must be accompanied by name of affiliated institution, date of term, and the signature of program/residency coordinator on institution letterhead. Orders will be billed at individual rate until proof of status is received. Foreign air speed delivery is included in all *Clinics* subscription prices. All prices are subject to change without notice. **POSTMASTER:** Send address changes to *Veterinary Clinics of North America: Exotic Animal Practice*, Elsevier Health Sciences Division, Subscription Customer Service, 3251 Riverport Lane, Maryland Heights,MO63043. **Customer Service: Telephone: 1-800-654-2452** (U.S. and Canada); **1-314-447-8871** (outside U.S. and Canada). **Fax: 1-314-447-8029. E-mail: journalscustomerservice-usa@elsevier.com** (for print support); **journalsonlinesupport-usa@elsevier.com** (for online support).

Reprints. For copies of 100 or more of articles in this publication, please contact the Commercial Reprints Department, Elsevier Inc., 360 Park Avenue South, New York, New York 10010-1710. Tel.: (212)-633-3813; Fax: (212)-633-1935; E-mail: reprints@elsevier.com.

Veterinary Clinics of North America: Exotic Animal Practice is covered in *MEDLINE/PubMed (Index Medicus)*.

Printed and bound by CPI Group (UK) Ltd, Croydon, CR0 4YY

Transferred to Digital Print 2012

Contributors

CONSULTING EDITOR

AGNES E. RUPLEY, DVM
Diplomate, American Board of Veterinary Practitioners–Avian Practice; Director and Chief Veterinarian, All Pets Medical & Laser Surgical Center, College Station, Texas

GUEST EDITOR

MARCY J. SOUZA, DVM, MPH
Diplomate, American Board of Veterinary Practitioners–Avian Practice; Diplomate, American College of Veterinary Preventive Medicine; Assistant Professor, Department of Comparative Medicine, College of Veterinary Medicine, The University of Tennessee, Knoxville, Tennessee

AUTHORS

SHANE BOYLAN, DVM
Staff Veterinarian, South Carolina Aquarium; Adjunct Faculty, Medical University of South Carolina; Adjunct Faculty, College of Charleston, Charleston, South Carolina

JULIE PAIGE BROWN, DVM
College of Veterinary Medicine, The University of Tennessee, Knoxville, Tennessee

ARMANDO G. BURGOS-RODRIGUEZ, DVM, ABVP-Avian
Staff Veterinarian, Caribbean Primate Research Center, Sabana Seca, Puerto Rico

L. RAND CARPENTER, DVM
Epidemiologist, Assistant State Public Health Veterinarian, Tennessee Department of Health, Communicable and Environmental Disease Services, Nashville, Tennessee

JOHN R. DUNN, DVM, PhD
Deputy State Epidemiologist, Tennessee Department of Health, Communicable and Environmental Disease Services, Nashville, Tennessee

ERIKA E. EVANS, DVM, MBA
Avian and Zoological Medicine Service, Department of Small Animal Clinical Sciences, College of Veterinary Medicine, The University of Tennessee, Knoxville, Tennessee

ALICE L. GREEN, MS, DVM
Public Health and Epidemiology Liaison, Office of Public Health Science, Food Safety and Inspection Service, United States Department of Agriculture, Minneapolis, Minnesota

VANESSA L. GRUNKEMEYER, DVM
Diplomate, American Board of Veterinary Practitioners-Avian; Department of Clinical Sciences, College of Veterinary Medicine, North Carolina State University, Raleigh, North Carolina

WILLIAM ALLEN HILL, DVM, MPH
Diplomate, American College of Laboratory Animal Medicine; Clinical Assistant
Professor, Department of Comparative Medicine, The University of Tennessee Institute
of Agriculture; Assistant Director, Office of Laboratory Animal Care, The University of
Tennessee, Knoxville, Tennessee

JÖRG MAYER, Drmedvet, MSc
Diplomate, American Board of Veterinary Practitioners-Exotic Companion Mammals;
Department of Small Animal Medicine and Surgery, College of Veterinary Medicine,
University of Georgia, Athens, Georgia

MARK A. MITCHELL, DVM, MS, PhD
Diplomate, European College of Zoological Medicine-Herpetology; Professor, Zoological
Medicine, Department of Veterinary Clinical Medicine, University of Illinois, College of
Veterinary Medicine, Urbana, Illinois

CHARLY PIGNON, DVM
Clinical Advisor; Head of the Exotics Medicine Service, Centre Hospitalier Universitaire
d'Alfort, Ecole Nationale Vétérinaire d'Alfort, Maisons-Alfort, France

EDWARD C. RAMSAY, DVM
Diplomate, American College of Zoological Medicine; Department of Small Animal
Clinical Sciences, College of Veterinary Medicine, The University of Tennessee,
Knoxville, Tennessee

MARCY J. SOUZA, DVM, MPH
Diplomate, American Board of Veterinary Practitioners–Avian Practice; Diplomate,
American College of Veterinary Preventive Medicine; Assistant Professor, Department of
Comparative Medicine, College of Veterinary Medicine, The University of Tennessee,
Knoxville, Tennessee

JULIA K. WHITTINGTON, DVM
Clinical Associate Professor; Service Chief, Zoological Medicine; Director, Wildlife
Medical Clinic, Department of Veterinary Clinical Medicine, University of Illinois, Urbana,
Illinois

Contents

Preface: Zoonoses, Public Health, and the Exotic Animal Practitioner   xi

Marcy J. Souza

One Health: Zoonoses in the Exotic Animal Practice   421

Marcy J. Souza

> Zoonoses make up approximately ¾ of today's emerging infectious diseases; many of these zoonoses come from exotic pets and wildlife. Recent outbreaks in humans associated with nondomestic animals include Sudden Acute Respiratory Syndrome, Ebola virus, salmonellosis, and monkeypox. Expanding human populations, increased exotic pet ownership and changes in climate may contribute to increased incidence of zoonoses. Education and preventive medicine practices can be applied by veterinarians and other health professionals to reduce the risk of contracting a zoonotic disease. The health of humans, animals, and the environment must be treated as a whole to prevent the transmission of zoonoses.

Zoonoses Associated with Fish   427

Shane Boylan

> The taxonomic group that composes the fishes is the most diverse group of vertebrates worldwide. The challenges of unique physiologics, a foreign environment, and many unknowns attract a passionate group of biologists and veterinarians. Economically, fishes have become vital as food, bait, and companion animals. Fishermen and fish handlers (processing plants) represent the historical human population exposed to fish zoonoses, but growth in aquaculture and aquarium hobbyists have led to an increase in published fish-borne zoonotic cases starting in the late 1950s that bloomed in the 1980s. Human physicians, particularly dermatologists and infectious disease specialists, are now more aware of fish-borne zoonoses, but they can be assisted with diagnosis when informed patients give more detailed histories with fish/water exposure.

Zoonotic Diseases Associated with Reptiles and Amphibians: An Update   439

Mark A. Mitchell

> Reptiles and amphibians are popular as pets. There are increased concerns among public health officials because of the zoonotic potential associated with these animals. Encounters with reptiles and amphibians are also on the rise in the laboratory setting and with wild animals; in both of these practices, there is also an increased likelihood for exposure to zoonotic pathogens. It is important that veterinarians

remain current with the literature as it relates to emerging and reemerging zoonotic diseases attributed to reptiles and amphibians so that they can protect themselves, their staff, and their clients from potential problems.

Zoonotic Diseases of Common Pet Birds: Psittacine, Passerine, and Columbiform Species   457

Erika E. Evans

Zoonotic transmission of disease from pet birds is uncommon, but there are some recognized dangers. Most notably, *Chlamydophila psittaci* can be transmitted from pet birds to humans. Allergic responses to pet birds, including pneumonitis and contact dermatitis, have also been documented. Bite wounds from pet birds are rarely reported but can cause trauma and develop infection. The other diseases discussed here are considered potential zoonotic diseases of pet birds because of either isolated reports of suspected but unconfirmed transmission to humans or from reports of wild conspecifics being reported to have the disease.

Zoonoses, Public Health, and the Backyard Poultry Flock   477

Vanessa L. Grunkemeyer

Raising a small flock of poultry for eggs, meat, and possibly companionship is becoming an increasingly popular hobby in the United States. Domestic chickens (*Gallus gallus, forma domestica*), turkeys (*Meleagris gallopavo, forma domestica*), and members of the family Anatidae including ducks, geese, and swans are commonly kept in these privately owned backyard flocks. Multiple bacterial, viral, fungal, and parasitic diseases which affect poultry are known zoonotic pathogens. This article reviews these zoonoses and gives recommendations for flock biosecurity, as well as for prevention of infection in both birds and humans. Diseases associated with other gallinaceous birds are only selectively discussed.

Public Health Concerns Associated with Care of Free-Living Birds   491

Julia K. Whittington

Free-living birds are not only susceptible to certain infectious diseases; wild bird populations serve as reservoirs of several important diseases of public health concern. Bacterial and viral diseases endemic in populations of free-living birds such as tuberculosis, avian influenza, arboviral infections, and enteropathogens have been classified as emerging or reemerging. Providing care to wild avian patients increases the opportunity for direct contact with infected birds and the possibility of transmission of infectious disease to human handlers. Awareness of disease potential is critical to disease monitoring of wild populations and will allow for the implementation of precautionary measures when working with wild avian species. Biosecurity measures designed to minimize risk must be evaluated by individual facilities.

Rabies Epidemiology, Risk Assessment, and Pre- and Post Exposure Vaccination   507

Alice L. Green, L. Rand Carpenter, and John R. Dunn

Rabies should always be considered in the differential diagnosis of a neurologic disease in a mammal with an unknown vaccination status. Public health veterinarians are available to assist in risk assessment as well as coordination of animal testing. This article discusses the pathogenesis of rabies and clinical presentation in several domestic species. Prevention, North American prevalence and distribution, exposure considerations, and post-exposure prophylaxis are also discussed. Veterinarians in private practice have an integral role in protection of people and domestic animals against rabies.

Zoonoses of Rabbits and Rodents   519

William Allen Hill and Julie Paige Brown

Millions of households in the US own rabbits or rodents, including hamsters, guinea pigs, and gerbils. Activities such as hunting and camping also involve human interactions with wild rabbits and rodents. In many environments, feral rabbits and rodents live in close proximity to humans, domesticated animals, and other wildlife. Education of rodent and rabbit owners and individuals with occupational or recreational exposures to these species is paramount to reduce the prevalence of zoonoses associated with rabbit and rodent exposure.

Zoonoses of Ferrets, Hedgehogs, and Sugar Gliders   533

Charly Pignon and Jörg Mayer

With urbanization, people live in close proximity to their pets. People often share their living quarters and furniture, and this proximity carries a new potential for pathogen transmission. In addition to the change in lifestyle with our pets, new exotic pets are being introduced to the pet industry regularly. Often, we are unfamiliar with specific clinical signs of diseases in these new exotic pets or the routes of transmission of pathogens for the particular species. This article reviews zoonoses that occur naturally in ferrets, hedgehogs, and sugar gliders, discussing the occurrence and clinical symptoms of these diseases in humans.

Zoonoses of Procyonids and Nondomestic Felids   551

Edward C. Ramsay

There are several important zoonotic diseases which can be acquired from procyonids, and nondomestic felids. *Baylisascaris procyonis*, the raccoon roundworm, is a common parasite of raccoons and can cause visceral, ocular, or neural larval migrans in people. Neural larval migrans can cause severe signs in individuals. Dermatophytosis and enteric pathogens are the most important zoonotic agents found in nondomestic felids. *Microsporum canis* infections can be spread from nondomestic felids to owners and veterinarians. *Toxoplasma gondii* can be potentially shed by infected felids, and human infections occurring during pregnancy can cause blindness in the fetus.

Zoonotic Diseases of Primates   557

Armando G. Burgos-Rodriguez

A zoonotic disease is transmissible from vertebrate animals to humans. This article focuses on pertinent zoonotic diseases that have to be taken into consideration when working with nonhuman primate (NHP) species. Many factors may influence the occurrence of these diseases. Human and NHPs share many similarities, not only anatomically but also physiologically. NHP are valuable models for many human infectious diseases; therefore, staff can be exposed to many potential pathogens. In general, the disease state of a primate can range from asymptomatic carrier to death from infection.

Index   577

FORTHCOMING ISSUES

January 2012

Mycobacteriosis
Miguel D. Saggese, DVM, PhD,
Guest Editor

May 2012

Pediatrics
Kristine Kuchinski, DVM, PhD,
Guest Editor

RECENT ISSUES

May 2011

The Exotic Animal Respiratory System
Susan E. Orosz, PhD, DVM, Dipl.
ABVP–Avian, Dipl. ECZM–Avian, and
Cathy A. Johnson-Delaney, DVM, Dipl.
ABVP–Avian and Exotic Companion
Mammal,
Guest Editors

January 2011

Analgesia and Pain Management
Joanne Paul-Murphy, DVM, Dipl. ACZM,
Guest Editor

September 2010

Advances and Updates in Internal Medicine
Kemba Marshall, DVM, DABVP–Avian,
Guest Editor

RELATED INTEREST

Veterinary Clinics of North America: Small Animal Practice (Volume 40, Issue 6, November 2010)
Current Topics in Canine and Feline Infectious Diseases
Stephen C. Barr, BVSc, MVS, PhD, *Guest Editor*

THE CLINICS ARE NOW AVAILABLE ONLINE!

Access your subscription at:
www.theclinics.com

Preface

Zoonoses, Public Health, and the Exotic Animal Practitioner

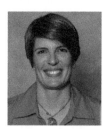

Marcy J. Souza, DVM, MPH, Dipl. ABVP–Avian, Dipl. ACVPM
Guest Editor

During my residency in Avian and Zoological Medicine at the University of Tennessee, people often asked me why I was pursuing a Masters degree in Public Health. I usually had two possible responses: 1) I like to torture myself and am going to have no life for the 3 years of my residency, so I may as well get as much out of it as possible; or the slightly longer version: 2) Do you realize that approximately three-fourths of today's emerging human pathogens come from animals? And, of these zoonoses, a large portion comes from exotic pets and wildlife! I would then proceed to run down the list of recent zoonotic epidemics and their associated animal reservoirs until they walked away or stopped paying attention.

Today, I commonly have veterinary students who are aspiring exotic/zoo/wildlife veterinarians come to me for advice. Some of the common questions are, "How can I get a residency?" or "How do I get your job?" There are usually two recommendations I make. First, I tell students that getting research experience during veterinary school is a great idea, regardless of what species they work on. Second, I recommend they pursue an MPH. I often have to give them explanation number 2 above so they understand the relevance to their professional goals.

Despite progress in human and veterinary medicine, pathogens are constantly evolving and staying one step in front of us. As the people of this world become more globally mobile and have closer, more frequent interactions with animals, the likelihood of future zoonotic epidemics seems inevitable. Additionally, changes in climate may alter the range of animal reservoirs or vectors, therefore changing the geographic distribution of current zoonoses. However, there are steps that can be taken to reduce the risk of contracting a zoonotic disease. These steps include not only quarantine and disinfection, but more importantly, education. All health care professionals, whether their patients are humans or animals, need to be engaged in education and prevention of zoonoses.

This issue of *Veterinary Clinics of North America: Exotic Animal Practice* has authors who are at the forefront of practicing, researching, and teaching exotic animal

doi:10.1016/j.cvex.2011.05.011
1094-9194/11/$ – see front matter © 2011 Elsevier Inc. All rights reserved.

and wildlife medicine. Each author was chosen (and thankfully accepted!) due to their specific expertise and interest. I am grateful to all of the authors that have helped make this issue possible. I am also grateful to Dr Agnes Rupley for asking me to edit an issue on the one subject I couldn't say "No" to and to John Vassallo for his help getting this issue organized and edited. I hope this issue will serve as an educational tool for veterinarians, and perhaps physicians, who want to know more about zoonoses and how to prevent them.

Marcy J. Souza, DVM, MPH, Dipl. ABVP–Avian, Dipl. ACVPM
Department of Comparative Medicine
University of Tennessee College of Veterinary Medicine
2407 River Drive
Knoxville, TN 37996, USA

E-mail address:
msouza@utk.edu

One Health: Zoonoses in the Exotic Animal Practice

Marcy J. Souza, DVM, MPH, Dipl. ABVP–Avian, Dipl. ACVPM

KEYWORDS

• Zoonoses • Exotic pets • Nontraditional pets • Wildlife
• Disease prevention

Recent outbreaks in humans associated with nondomestic animal species include Sudden Acute Respiratory Syndrome (SARS), Ebola virus, salmonellosis, and monkeypox. Animals may act as sentinels for human health. Expanding human populations and encroachment on habitats may increase exposure to zoonotic agents. Education and preventive medicine practices can be applied to reduce the risk of contracting a zoonotic disease. The health of humans, animals, and the environment must be treated as a whole to prevent the transmission of zoonoses.

ZOONOSES

Zoonoses are estimated to make up 75% of today's emerging infectious diseases.[1] Many of these zoonoses are carried by exotic pets or wildlife species,[2] and recent outbreaks in humans associated with nondomestic species include Sudden Acute Respiratory Syndrome (SARS),[3] Ebola virus,[4] salmonellosis,[5] and monkeypox.[6,7] Some of these infectious agents can cause disease in animals, and these animals may act as sentinels for human health. Expanding human populations and subsequent encroachment on habitats of reservoir species of zoonoses, increased trade in and ownership of "exotic" pets, and changes in climate will likely lead to increased exposure to zoonotic agents. Veterinarians could be held legally responsible for the transmission of zoonoses to staff or clients. Education and preventive medicine practices can be applied to reduce the risk of contracting a zoonotic disease by veterinarians, their staff, or owners of exotic pets. The health of humans, animals, and the environment are linked and must be treated as a whole to prevent the transmission of zoonoses and increase our understanding of the concept of "One Health."

RECENT EPIDEMICS

Numerous recent epidemics have been associated with exotic pets or wildlife species including SARS, Ebola, salmonellosis, and monkeypox. Morbidity and mortality in humans varies with each etiologic agent; animals can sometimes also be affected

Department of Comparative Medicine, University of Tennessee College of Veterinary Medicine, Knoxville, TN 37996, USA
E-mail address: msouza@utk.edu

Vet Clin Exot Anim 14 (2011) 421–426
doi:10.1016/j.cvex.2011.05.007
1094-9194/11/$ – see front matter © 2011 Elsevier Inc. All rights reserved.

with disease. More dangerous, though, reservoir species may be asymptomatic and provide no outward sign that they are potential sources of zoonotic agents. Transmission and case identification often results in large scale costly investigations to determine the source of an outbreak and apply steps to reduce further spread of disease.

In February 2003, an outbreak of respiratory disease was recognized in approximately a dozen people in a Hong Kong hotel. The infection, later determined to be caused by a novel coronavirus, eventually led to 8,096 human cases with 774 deaths in 26 countries worldwide.[8] Many of the early cases occurred in the Guangdong province of China and were associated with animal or food handling; later cases were associated with direct contact with an infected human. Himalayan palm civets (*Paguma larvata*) found in live animal markets and wild fruit bats have both been implicated as possible reservoirs of SARS-like coronaviruses.[3,9] There have been no reports of illness in civets or bats associated with these coronaviruses; however, nonhuman primates develop illness when experimentally infected.[8]

Numerous outbreaks of Ebola have occurred in humans in Central Africa since the 1970s; mortality is typically high, but variable.[10] Many outbreaks have been associated with exposure to nonhuman primates, but Ebola virus also causes significant mortality in gorillas (*Gorilla gorilla*) and chimpanzees (*Pan troglodytes*).[10,11] A few outbreaks were also associated with exposure to duikers and monkeys.[10] Fruit bats have recently been implicated as reservoirs for Ebola virus but do not develop disease.[4] Although Ebola virus infection is rare outside of Africa, quarantine procedures must still be followed to avoid the importation of infected animals such as occurred with imported primates for laboratories in Virginia and Texas.[12,13] The Centers for Disease Control and Prevention (CDC) regulate importation and quarantine of all nonhuman primates, as well as any other animal that may carry zoonotic pathogens.[14]

Historically, salmonellosis from exotic animals has most commonly been associated with exposure to reptiles, but a recent outbreak in 2009 was associated with exposure to aquatic frogs.[5] The outbreak was caused by *Salmonella* Typhimurium and the organism was isolated from 85 people in 31 states of the USA. No deaths were reported, but numerous people required hospitalization. An investigation determined that exposure to African dwarf frogs (*Hymenochyrus spp*) was associated with infection, and the organism was isolated from animals, samples from tanks where pet frogs were housed, and breeder facilities. Similar to reptiles, amphibians can be asymptomatic carriers of *Salmonella*. The CDC concluded that educational material addressing *Salmonella* exposure from reptiles should also include amphibians as possible sources of the organism.[15]

In 2003, an outbreak of monkeypox (orthopoxvirus) was linked to exposure to pet prairie dogs (*Cynomus sp*) in the US. Eighty-one human cases were reported in 6 states.[6,7] Numerous species of African rodents that had been imported for the pet trade were found to be positive for the monkeypox virus associated with the outbreak. Imported rodents had been commingled with prairie dogs that were eventually sold as pets. One study showed that prairie dogs do develop disease and suffer mortality when infected with monkeypox.[16] CDC issued guidance on the quarantine and euthanasia of animals in the infected shipment as well as other exposed animals, particularly prairie dogs.[17]

CONTRIBUTING FACTORS

Numerous factors may contribute to the continued increasing exposure to zoonoses from wildlife and exotic pets.[18] Some of these factors include: a continually growing and globalized human population, increased exotic pet ownership, and changes in climate that affect wildlife and vector distribution.

As human populations continue to increase, more people will move into areas that have not previously been inhabited and alter the environment to suit their purposes, whether for housing or agriculture; interactions with native wildlife and invertebrate vectors of disease will increase as a result.[19,20] One study found that increased interactions with wildlife occurred in suburban and exurban communities, while fewer interactions occurred in more densely populated communities.[21] Interactions may lead to increased exposure to zoonotic pathogens through direct contact with animals, contact with infected urine, feces, pelts or a carcass, or exposure to vectors such as ticks or fleas. Zooanthroponotic pathogen (those passed from humans to animals) exposure to animals may also increase with these interactions.[22] Additionally, as humans move into previously uninhabited areas, consumption of native wildlife may increase leading to increased exposure to zoonotic agents. Historically, tularemia was associated with rabbit hunting, and now Ebola virus outbreaks are associated with the bush meat trade in Africa.[23] Larger human populations will require increasingly larger amounts of protein for sustenance, and some of this protein will undoubtedly come from wildlife. Finally, because of increased ease of international travel and globalization of cultures, humans, animals, and pathogens can travel the globe quickly allowing diseases to spread rapidly worldwide.[24]

Although dogs and cats are still the largest population of pets in the US, the American Veterinary Medical Association reports that ownership has increased from 2001 to 2007 for the following other types of pets: fish, ferrets, rabbits, hamsters, guinea pigs, other rodents (not specifically identified), turtles, snakes, and lizards.[25] A category titled "all others" also increased from 2001 to 2007, but the specific animals included in this category were not listed. The total number of birds kept as pets has increased, but the number of households owning birds decreased in the same time period. In general, the number of households with pets other than dogs and cats is increasing. Depending on the country of origin of these exotic pets, and what importation and quarantine procedures are performed, exotic pets may carry zoonoses that have not previously been identified in that particular geographic area[19]; numerous outbreaks of zoonoses have been associated with the legal and illegal importation of animals in the pet trade.[20] The identification of monkeypox in a population of pet prairie dogs in the midwestern US is an excellent example of how non-native exotic rodents that were carrying a zoonotic agent uncommon to the US transmitted the virus to native rodents in the pet trade; no human cases were directly caused by the non-native exotic rodents.[6]

Global climate change is occurring and is unlikely to slow without significant measures by humans.[26] These climate changes are not only expected to directly affect humans through more severe and prolonged weather events, but also by changing the home range of wildlife species and vectors of disease, such as ticks, and altering the time when a disease can typically be transmitted to humans. One recent study predicts that the range of *Ixodes scapularis*, the primary tick that transmits the etiologic agent of Lyme disease in the US, will noticeably expand in the next two decades with the predicted rate of climate change; this change in range of the vector species will also affect the geographic distribution of the disease in humans and animals, such as dogs.[27] Another paper suggests that the current ranges of plague and tularemia are likely to shift north due to changes in range of host rodent species, although the changes will likely be subtle.[28] Prevalence, intensity, and geographic distribution of disease due to some helminths are also expected to change with changes in climate.[29] Finally, milder winters and earlier springs may lead to alterations in the typical transmission period of some vector borne diseases. For example, West Nile virus, which typically peaks in late summer, could be transmitted earlier in the year leading to a higher incidence of disease in humans earlier in the year.[26] The total effects of climate change on zoonotic disease transmission and distribution is still unknown, and there are many factors that complicate predictions.[26] Regardless of the specifics, alterations in disease distribution and transmission are expected as a result of changes in climate.

LEGAL IMPLICATIONS

Veterinarians, as well as physicians and other health care professionals, have a responsibility to protect human health. A recent paper reports several scenarios where a veterinarian could potentially breach their professional duty and be subject to litigation.[30] These scenarios include: (1) failure to recommend preventive measures to owners of animals with zoonotic diseases, (2) failure to advise clients on the dangers of exotic pets, and (3) failure to advise clients to seek care from a physician when appropriate. Veterinarians, as members of any community's health care team, must not only treat animals, but also play a role in the prevention of zoonoses in humans. Educational materials and counseling should be provided to pet owners regarding zoonoses and how to prevent their transmission.

Veterinarians, physicians, and other health care professionals must also increase communication between each other regarding zoonoses. A recent study found that 97% of veterinarians rarely or never contacted physicians regarding animal aspects of zoonoses or transmission of zoonoses to an individual person with HIV/AIDS.[31] In the same study, 100% of physicians rarely or never contacted a veterinarian regarding the animal aspects of zoonoses transmission or transmission of zoonoses to an individual HIV/AIDS patient. All health professionals must communicate and play a role in human and animal health in order to facilitate the concept of "One Health."

Finally, veterinarians must take steps to prevent zoonoses in the personnel under their supervision. These steps may include having standard operating procedures in place to prevent zoonoses, disinfecting contaminated areas, and providing education for staff regarding disease prevention. Specific guidelines regarding disease prevention are available in the Compendium of Veterinary Standard Precautions for Zoonotic Disease Prevention in Veterinary Personnel.[32] Many of these recommendations can also be given to pet owners that are caring for a sick animal at home.

CONCLUSIONS

Human, animal, and environmental health are intertwined and must all be considered when dealing with zoonotic diseases. With expanding human populations, increased exotic pet ownership, and changes in climate, human exposure to zoonotic agents will continue and likely increase. Veterinarians must not only treat animals with zoonoses, but also play a role in the prevention of zoonoses in humans. Veterinarians should work with physicians to provide education and preventive measures to humans in order to reduce the likelihood of zoonoses transmission.

ACKNOWLEDGMENTS

Special thanks to Dr John New for reviewing this manuscript and providing guidance to me in veterinary public health.

REFERENCES

1. Taylor LH, Latham SM, Woolhouse ME. Risk factors for human disease emergence. Philos Trans R Soc Lond B Biol Sci 2001;356(1411):983–9.
2. Jones KE, Patel NG, Levy MA, et al. Global trends in emerging infectious diseases. Nature 2008;451:990–3.
3. Guan Y, Zheng BJ, He YQ, et al. Isolation and characterization of viruses related to the SARS coronavirus from animals in southern China. Science 2003;302:276–8.
4. Leroy EM, Kumulungui B, Pourrut X, et al. Fruit bats as reservoirs of Ebola virus. Nature 2005;438:575–6.
5. Centers for Disease Control and Prevention. Multistate outbreak of human Salmonella typhimurium infections associated with aquatic frogs - United States, 2009. MMWR Morb Mortal Wkly Rep 2010;58:1433–6.
6. Centers for Disease Control and Prevention. Multistate outbreak of monkeypox–Illinois, Indiana, and Wisconsin, 2003a. MMWR Morb Mortal Wkly Rep 2003;52:537–40.
7. Centers for Disease Control and Prevention. Update: Multistate outbreak of monkey-pox–Illinois, Indiana, Kansas, Missouri, Ohio, and Wisconsin, 2003. MMWR Morb Mortal Wkly Rep 2003;52:616–8.
8. Skowronski DM, Astell C, Brunham RC, et al. Severe acute respiratory syndrome (SARS): a year in review. Annu Rev Med 2005;56:357–81.
9. Li W, Shi Z, Yu M, et al. Bats are natural reservoirs of SARS-like coronaviruses. Science 2005;310:676–79.
10. Leroy EM, Epelboin A, Mondonge V, et al. Human Ebola outbreak resulting from direct exposure to fruit bats in Luebo, Democratic Republic of Congo, 2007. Vector Borne Zoonotic Dis 2009;9:723–8.
11. Huijbregts B, De Wachter P, Sosthene L, et al. Ebola and the decline of gorilla Gorilla gorilla and chimpanzee Pan troglodytes populations in Minkebe Forest, north-eastern Gabon. Oryx 2003;37:437–43.
12. Centers for Disease Control and Prevention (CDC). Ebola virus infections in imported primates--Virginia, 1989. MMWR Morb Mortal Wkly Rep 1989;38:831 8.
13. Centers for Disease Control and Prevention (CDC). Ebola-Reston virus infection among quarantine nonhuman primates--Texas, 1996. MMWR Morb Mortal Wkly Rep 1996;45:314–6.
14. Centers for Disease Contol and Prevention (CDC). Importing Animals (including pets) and Animal Products. Available at: http://www.cdc.gov/animalimportation/. Accessed January 17, 2011.
15. Centers for Disease Contol and Prevention (CDC). Investigation update: outbreak of human Salmonella Typhimurium infections associated with contact with water frogs. Available at: http://www.cdc.gov/salmonella/typh1209/. Accessed January 17, 2011.
16. Guarner J, Johnson BJ, Paddock CD, et al. Monkeypox transmission and pathogenesis in prairie dogs. Emerg Infect Dis 2004;10:426–31.
17. Centers for Disease Control and Prevention (CDC). Questions and Answers About Monkeypox. Available at: http://www.cdc.gov/ncidod/monkeypox/qa.htm. Accessed January 17, 2011.
18. Cutler SJ, Fooks AR, van der Poel WH. Public health threat of new, reemerging, and neglected zoonoses in the industrialized world. Emerg Infect Dis 2010;16:1–7.
19. Chomel BB, Belotto A, Meslin FX. Wildlife, exotic pets, and emerging zoonoses. Emerg Infect Dis 2007;13:6–11.

20. Greger M. The human/animal interface: emergence and resurgence of zoonotic infectious diseases. Crit Rev Microbiol 2007;33:243–99.

21. Kretser HE, Sullivan PJ, Knuth BA. Housing density as an indicator of spatial patterns of reported human-wildlife interactions in Northern New York. Landscape Urban Plann 2008;84:282–92.

22. Epstein JH, Price JT. The significant but understudied impact of pathogen transmission from humans to animals. Mt Sinai J Med 2009;76:448–55.

23. Karesh WB, Noble E. The bushmeat trade: increased opportunities for transmission of zoonotic disease. Mt Sinai J Med 2009;76:429–34.

24. Brown C. Emerging zoonoses and pathogens of public health significance—an overview. Rev Sci Tech 2004;23:435–42.

25. American Veterinary Medical Association. US pet ownership—2007. Available at: http://www.avma.org/reference/marketstats/ownership.asp. Accessed December 29, 2010.

26. Greer A, Ng V, Fisman D. Climate change and infectious diseases in North America: the road ahead. CMAJ 2008;178:715–22.

27. Ogden NH, Maarouf A, Barker IK, et al. Climate change and the potential for range expansion of the Lyme disease vector Ixodes scapularis in Canada. Int J Parasitol 2006;36:63–70.

28. Nakazawa Y, Williams R, Peterson AT, et al. Climate change effects of plague and tularemia in the United States. Vector Borne Zoonotic Dis 2007;7:529–40.

29. Mas-Coma S, Valero MA, Bargues MD. Effects of climate change on animal and zoonotic helminthiases. Rev Sci Tech 2008;27:443–57.

30. Babcock S, Marsh AE, Lin J, et al. Legal implications of zoonoses for clinical veterinarians. J Amer Vet Med Assoc 2008;233:1556–62.

31. Hill WA, Petty G, Erwin P, et al. Prevention of zoonoses among companion animal owners infected with HIV/AIDS: a survey of Tennessee veterinarian and physician attitudes, knowledge, and practices. J Amer Vet Med Assoc, in press.

32. National Association of State Public Health Veterinarians (NASPHV). Compendium of veterinary standard precautions for zoonotic disease prevention in veterinary personnel. Available at: http://www.nasphv.org/Documents/VeterinaryPrecautions.pdf. Accessed January 2, 2011.

Zoonoses Associated with Fish

Shane Boylan, DVM[a,b,c,]*

KEYWORDS

- Fish • Zoonoses • Atypical mycobacteria • Vibrio
- Edwardsiella • Erysipelothrix • *S iniae*

The taxonomic group that composes the fishes is the most diverse group of vertebrates worldwide. The challenges of unique physiologies, a foreign environment, and many unknowns attract a passionate group of biologists and veterinarians. Economically, fishes have become vital as food, bait, and companion animals. Fishermen and fish handlers (processing plants) represent the historical human population exposed to fish zoonoses, but growth in aquaculture and aquarium hobbyists have led to an increase in published fish-borne zoonotic cases starting in the late 1950s that bloomed in the 1980s.[1–9] Human physicians, particularly dermatologists and infectious disease specialists, are now more aware of fish-borne zoonoses, but they can be assisted with diagnosis when informed patients give more detailed histories with fish/water exposure.[8]

One role of the veterinarian is to inform clients about the potential risks of zoonotic disease. While fish-borne zoonoses are rare, the attention they have received in the past few decades has increased due to an overall focus on zoonotic diseases like avian influenza, tick-borne illness, bovine spongiform encephalopathy (BSE), and West Nile virus.[8,10] A recent review of aquatic zoonoses is available.[11] Fortunately, the diversity of fish-borne zoonotic pathogens is restricted to a small number of opportunistic bacterial pathogens. The disease triad of pathogen, host, and environment must always be considered when dealing with fish-borne zoonoses. Immune-compromised veterinarians exposing themselves to heavy infective doses of a pathogen may find themselves with an infection of a novel bacteria or fungus not previously described in the medical literature. Human immunodeficiency virus has demonstrated that many organisms previously considered innocuous can become potentially life threatening when the immune system is altered.[12,13] Fish-borne viral zoonoses have yet to be diagnosed, although some viruses show a tremendous capacity to jump between species in the aquatic environment.[14]

---

a South Carolina Aquarium, Charleston, SC, USA
b Medical University of South Carolina, Charleston, SC, USA
c College of Charleston, Charleston, SC, USA
* South Carolina Aquarium, 100 Aquarium Wharf, Charleston, SC 29401.
E-mail address: sboylan@scaquarium.org

Vet Clin Exot Anim 14 (2011) 427–438
doi:10.1016/j.cvex.2011.05.003
1094-9194/11/$ – see front matter © 2011 Elsevier Inc. All rights reserved.

PROTOZOA AND PARASITES

Protozoal pathogens are arguably the most prevalent and damaging form of disease in ornamental piscine aquaculture.[15] Zoonotic protozoal fish pathogens are not reported in the literature, although protozoal organisms like *Cryptosporidium* spp, *Giardia lamblia*, *Balantidium* spp, malarial trypanosomes, and *Toxoplasma gondii* are found in aquatic environments where humans can be potentially exposed.[16,17]

Fish-borne parasitic zoonoses are not a typical concern for the veterinarian as part of their practice. Cestodiasis, trematodiasis, pentastomiasis, and nematodiasis are conditions that most aquatic veterinarians treat in their aquatic patients, but the clinician should always remember that a few of these parasites may use humans as a definitive, intermediate, or paratenic host. The clinician should be aware of the complex life cycles of these parasites and the clinical concerns they represent to both animal and human, particularly in food aquaculture. Consumption of raw, under-cooked, undersalted, or insufficiently pickled fish meats is the primary route of fish parasite transmission to humans.[18,19] Cultural and socioeconomical factors predispose certain people to infection with the majority of fish-borne parasitic zoonoses occurring in lower-income countries.[18,20] The movement of aquaculture species has also led to the introduction of zoonotic parasites where medical surveillance and diagnosis for these pathogens are usually underdeveloped.[18,19] Gnathostomasis is an example where a helminth parasite is expanding its range due to human dietary and aquaculture practices.[19] Even the immigration/emigration of infected people, who act as definite hosts with fecal egg shedding, have increased the distribution of several parasites like clonorchis/opisthorchis liver flukes.[18,20,21]

In humans, the majority of fish-borne zoonotic parasites show few clinical symptoms unless parasite burdens are high. Biliary and hepatic lesions are common manifestations with hepatic trematode infections. Intestinal, pancreatic, and even bronchial disease are clinical symptoms of parasites that use the gastrointestinal system, like anisakiid nematodes, intestinal flukes, and diphyllobothriid cestodes.[18,19] Cancerous or precancerous growths have also been associated with infections of fish-borne parasite zoonoses in humans.[18,21] Liver fluke infections produce hepatic hyperplasia that may be diagnosed as cholangiohepatic carcinomas.[21,22] In the Pacific Northwest of the United States, the zoonotic intestinal fluke *Nanophyetus salmincola* causes "salmon poisoning" in canids by transmitting the rickettsia *Neorickettsia helmintheca*.[18] Oddly, the fluke causes gastrointestinal disease in humans without apparent pathology contribution by the rickettsia.[18] Although the majority of zoonotic fish parasite life cycles cannot be established in indoor environments, veterinarians working with outdoor aquaculture should be vigilant for these rare zoonotic parasites where life cycles may be completed. Even in ornamental aquaculture, predatory wildlife may spread parasites to areas of food aquaculture that could lead to human zoonoses. Veterinarians should assist in efforts to reduce exposure of all cultured fish to native wildlife, which can sustain significant disease and act as vectors for parasite transmission. Proper disposal of fish carcasses, enclosures that keep out predators, proper handling of waste water, and other containment practices may protect both cultured fish and wildlife. The nematode *Anguicolla crassus* (Asia) is one example of a foreign nematode that is now established in wild eel populations in North America and Europe as a result of possible contamination by introduced aqua-cultured animals.[23,24] Although *Anguicolla crassus* nematodes are not zoonotic, the example reveals how introduced fish parasites can harm both aquaculture and native wildlife.[25]

FUNGI

To the author's knowledge, fish-borne zoonotic fungal pathogens have not been reported in the literature. Since many fungi are opportunistic pathogens, the potential exists that fishes or aquatic fomites with heavy infectious burdens could cause a human infection through a puncture, open wound, or similar route. The fungal genus *Exophilia* includes species that are established as fish and mammalian pathogens.[26–29]

BACTERIA

Bacteria are the main fish-borne zoonotic agents that should concern the veterinary clinician. Infection is typically acquired through abrasions, cuts, or penetrating wounds in the skin when handling infected fish or fomites (water). Recirculating systems often have high organic loads that are an excellent growth media for many bacteria. Most of the bacteria described next are often present even when clinical signs are absent in fish, so personal protection equipment (PPE) such as gloves should always be worn. The majority of these bacterial pathogens are gram negative, although certain gram-positive bacteria are medically relevant.

Mycobacterium

The most important fish-borne zoonotic bacterial agent is atypical mycobacteriosis.[30] This group of gram-positive, aerobic, non–spore-forming, acid-fast positive, nonmotile rods are ubiquitous in both marine and freshwater environments.[31] Atypical mycobacteria are different from their more familiar cousins (*Mycobacterium tuberculosis, M bovis, M avium*) because they are slow-growing, mildly psychrophilic to mesophilic environmental organisms that typically cause infections in the extremities of humans where temperatures are cooler than 33°C (91°F).[5] There are nearly 120 species of *Mycobacteria,* with *M marinum, M fortuitum,* and *M ulcerans* discussed most commonly as fish-borne zoonoses.[31–34]

Clinical disease is known by a variety of monikers, including "fish handler's disease," "tank granuloma," and "fish fancier's finger." Infection severity ranges from self-limiting to moderate dermatitis requiring treatment.[33,34] Immunocompromised patients with atypical mycobacteriosis can progress into systemic infections that are fatal.[5,35] Lesions typically present as less than 2-cm-diameter, nodular, reddened swellings in the skin and joints of the extremities[3,6,33,34] (**Fig. 1**). The size, tenderness, and number of swellings slowly increase over weeks to months, when discomfort causes patients to seek medical attention.[5,34] Yellowish exudates can sometimes be expressed from these lesions where acid-fast cytology may reveal the presence of the organisms.[3,7] Patients need to include a possible history of exposure to water and/or fish since other differentials may be explored before atypical mycobacteriosis is even considered by the physician.[34] Many patients are often misdiagnosed and treated with topical/oral antibiotics, antifungals, or steroids that have no effect or actually exacerbate the condition (steroids).[3,5,6,34] Definitive diagnosis usually requires a positive polymerase chain reaction (PCR) and biopsy/aspiration cultures with sensitivities. Initial therapies vary but many patients are put on a treatment of 2 antibiotics, usually rifampin and minocycline/ethambutol.[33,34] Cultures and sensitivities can take several weeks due to the slow-growing nature of the bacteria, and antibiotic therapy is often changed since resistance to initial therapy is not uncommon[2,3,6,7,33] (Shane Boylan, Charleston, SC, personal communication, December 2010). Antibiotic therapy typically lasts months with routine blood analysis conducted to monitor the liver and kidneys. In severe cases, surgical debridement, cryotherapy, x-ray therapy, and electrodesiccation may be necessary to facilitate clearance.[33]

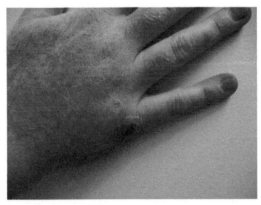

Fig. 1. Red, circular lesion on the hand from atypical mycobacteriosis infection. (*Courtesy of* Gregory A. Lewbart, MS, VMD, Raleigh, NC.)

Disinfection of materials exposed to atypical mycobacteria can be challenging. Biofilms and thick cell walls make atypical mycobacteria resistant to the common forms of aquatic disinfection of quaternary ammonia compounds and dilute sodium hypochlorite (Bleach).[36,37] Even gluteraldehyde and new powerful oxidants require mechanical scrubbing to remove biofilms to effectively kill atypical mycobacteria.[36,38] Phenols, high concentrations of alcohol, and strong sodium chlorite solutions are effective for disinfection.[39] The mycobacteria, *M chelonae* and *M avium-intracellulare*, can commonly be cultured from chlorinated tap water systems and sterilized endoscopy equipment.[37,40–42] Disposal of contaminated aquarium water varies by location and local health authorities should be contacted regarding specific regulations.

Low stomach pH and higher body temperatures usually prevent oral transmission of atypical mycobacteria in healthy humans, however, the fecal-oral route and shedding from cutaneous lesions are usually considered the primary routes of bacteria dispersal among fish.[43,44] Many fishes remain asymptomatic carriers/ shedders for long periods of time. Clinical signs vary but chronic infections typically include skin ulceration and loss of body condition despite eating with exophthalmia, ascites, and possibly micro/macro granulomas. Anyone dealing with sygnathid aquaculture (seahorses, pipefish) should always wear PPE as these fish are highly susceptible to mycobacteria infection (**Fig. 2**). Kinyoun carbol fuceshin stains (Jorgensen Laboratories Inc, Loveland, CO, USA) of tissue smears of various organs can be used to identify acid fast positive rods which when combined with clinical signs of emaciation and visceral granulomas, put atypical mycobacteriosis as the most likely differential (**Fig. 3**). This kind of rapid, counter-top cytological test can give the veterinary clinician immediate guidance while they wait for send-off tests like histopathology, PCR, and cultures.

Streptococcus iniae

Another gram positive fish-borne zoonotic bacterium is *Streptococcus iniae* which was first described in a captive Amazon River dolphin, *Inia geofrensis*.[45,46] *Streptococcus iniae* has been found to infect several species of commercially valuable fish including tilapia (*Oreochromis* spp, *Tilapia* spp, and *Sarotherodon* spp), channel catfish (*Ictalurus punctatus*), and hybrid striped bass (*Morone* spp).[47–49] Clinical signs

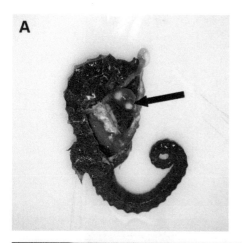

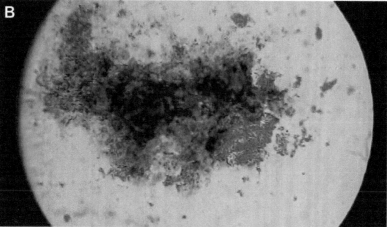

Fig. 2. (*A*) Large, coelomic granulomas in a *Hippocampus erectus* that were positive for acid fast rods (*B*). (*Courtesy of* Shane Boylan, DVM, Charleston, SC.)

in fish include the loss of orientation, petechial hemorrhages, exophthalmia, and corneal hypopyon.[47,48] In humans, handling of live or recently killed infected fish can produce cellulitis of the hand or endocarditis, meningitis, and arthritis in severe systemic infections.[45,50–52] Culture of *S iniae* is best achieved from brain tissue of affected fish where most other bacterial pathogens are best isolated from kidney cultures.[49,50]

Erysipelothrix rhusiopathiae

The last gram-positive bacterium associated with fish-borne zoonoses is *Erysipelothrix rhusiopathiae*. This pathogen is associated with disease in marine mammals where it causes systemic or rhomboid skin disease, possibly killing cetaceans with acute septicemia.[53] No reports of actual disease occur in fish, and the bacteria are commonly found in fishes' cutaneous mucus.[54] Like the majority of fish-borne bacterial zoonoses, infection occurs when exposed wounds encounter bacteria in fish mucus usually during handling of live or dead fish. Human

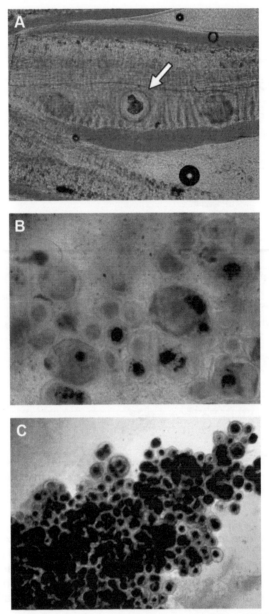

Fig. 3. Wet mount squash preparations of gill (*A*), intestine (*B*), and kidney (*C*) tissue with numerous microgranulomas that were acid-fast positive in an Atlantic bumper (*Chloroscombrus chrysurus*). (*Courtesy of* Shane Boylan, DVM, Charleston, SC.)

clinical symptoms include localized infections of the extremities, diffuse cutaneous infections, and systemic disease including endocarditis.[55,56] *Erysipelothrix rhusiopathiae* is resistant to freezing so handlers of frozen fish as food should also wear appropriate gloves.

Aeromonas and Vibrio

Gram-negative bacteria are the most common microbial pathogens of fish. The Aeromonads are ubiquitous gram negative, usually freshwater, motile rods that can cause opportunistic infection in numerous fish species. *Aeromonas hydrophila* is the most commonly reported species that possesses zoonotic potential although *A sobria* and *A caviae* have also been reported.[57–59] Usually environmental stressors or coinfection with another agent is required for a piscine infection with *A hydrophila*. Fish lesions are consistent with sepsis including petechia in the skin and fins, ulcerations and erythema of the skin, anorexia, exophthalmia, and ascites.[45,58] Waters with high nutrient levels can create *Aeromonas* spp blooms that could be infectious to humans through wounds or ingestion; infections in humans are rare and typically involve immune suppression. *Aeromonas salmonicida*, a nonmotile facultative aerobic rod, is an obligate fish pathogen in both freshwater and marine fish. Infection is often described as "fish furunculosis" and is a well-known disease among salmonid aquaculture and cyprinid hobbyists (koi and goldfish).[58] *Aeromonas salmonicida* has not appeared in the medical literature as a zoonotic agent although it is often discussed with fish zoonoses.[11,60]

Vibrio spp are considered the marine analog of the Aeromonads, but both bacterial genera have marine and freshwater members.[61] Like *Aeromonas* spp, *Vibrio* spp infection can remain asymptomatic until environmental stressors produce disease. Clinical signs in fish are consistent with sepsis including anorexia, ulcerations, exophthalmia, and petechia/erythema.[62] The similarities between *Vibrio* spp and *Aeromonas* spp extend to their range of infectivity in fish and aquatic invertebrates.[49,62] Human infections with *V cholerae*, *V damselae* (*Photobacterium damselae*), *V parahaemolyticus*, *V vulnificusare* (*V vulnificus*), *V harveyi* (*V carchariae*), *V fluvialis*, *V mimicus*, *V metschnikovii*, *V hollisae* (*Grimontia hollisae*), and *V alginolyticus* occur occasionally through skin wounds or more commonly through ingestion of infected shellfish.[8,61–63]

Edwardsiella

Edwardsiella tarda is a gram negative, motile, facultative anaerobic rod that is a zoonotic pathogen found in numerous species of freshwater fish. Although not as devastating to the United States channel catfish industry as *E ictaluri*, *E tarda* causes clinical signs including myonecrosis, organ necrosis, hepatic abscesses, coelomitis, hypopyon, hemorrhage, ascites, ulceration/hemorrhage, and necrosis of the lateral line system.[64] Human infections most often occur with the consumption of infected tissue/water resulting in gastroenteritis although exposure to open wounds with immune suppression can cause significant cellulitis, myconecrosis, and sepsis.[9,57,65–67]

Salmonella and others

Salmonella spp (Enterobacteriaceae) bacteria are zoonotic, gram-negative rods classically associated with freshwater aquatic turtles and amphibians.[68,69] The author is unaware of any fish salmonellosis reports despite the abundance of the organism in aquatic environments. Since many outdoor ornamental fish ponds have wild reptiles and amphibians present, the veterinarian should always relay this potential threat to their clients. Piscine francisellosis is a recently reported fish disease with the potential for zoonosis due to the close homology of fish isolates to the deadly mammalian pathogen, *Francisella tularensis*, although no human infections have been reported.[70] Nile tilapia, *Oreochromis niloticus*, with francisellosis show signs including erratic swimming, exophthalmia, and anorexia.[70,71] Other bacteria associated with water that may be remotely associated with fish-borne zoonoses are Enterobacteriacae (Citrobacter spp, Serratia spp), Pseudomonas spp, Shigella spp, Staphlococcus spp, Listeria spp, and Clostridium spp.[11,60]

PREVENTION OF DISEASE

For the veterinarian, nearly every zoonotic bacteria gains access through disruption of the innate immune system, primarily through puncture, cuts, scrapes, abrasions, or sores in the skin. Oral ingestion of fish-borne zoonotic agents has been briefly discussed here; numerous articles review the topic in more detail with regard to food safety.[72,73] Aquaculture systems range in design from home hobbyist aquaria, to flow through raceways, to huge acre ponds, but they all have nutrient-rich waters that benefit bacterial proliferation. Numerous studies have been conducted on proper chemical disinfection of contaminated surfaces; contact time, proper safe handling of disinfectants, and accurate dosing of disinfectants should be emphasized as part of the veterinarian-client-patient relationship. Ironically, one of the best disinfection methods for exposed surfaces is simple dessication/drying. Even with biofilms, significant exposure to drying environments like direct sunlight when given enough time, will completely kill aquatic pathogens including the resistant atypical mycobacteria.

As a matter of practice, most aquatic clinicians have suffered numerous puncture wounds/bites without incident and therefore may have a cavalier attitude toward zoonoses until they experience an infection themselves or know someone who has. Veterinarians, their staff, and clients should always safeguard themselves by reducing exposure of open cuts and abrasions to water. Disposable gloves can protect fish handlers during the multitude of tasks that allow fish mucus/tissue/waste to contact skin including: fish processing for food, veterinary exams, surgeries, vaccination, or husbandry procedures. Tissue glue, Vasoline®, betadine gels, and topical ointments like triple antibiotic and silver sulfadiazine can be applied over open surface wounds when water contact is unavoidable; however, wearing disposable gloves is still recommended. Deep puncture trauma should be thoroughly flushed with some form of disinfectant (hydrogen peroxide, alcohol, betadine, chlorhexidine) followed by sterile saline or water soon after injury occurs. Deep puncture wounds represent the greatest risk and should receive medical attention.

Veterinarians have an obligation to inform clients and act by example with proper use of PPE. Clients should be informed about zoonoses when working with fish without overdramatizing the risks. Emphasis should be placed on protecting the extremities and avoiding exposure during immune suppression. If a possible fish-borne zoonosis is suspected, an informed client will be able to give a more thorough history to their physician. Veterinarians must communicate with clients, staff, and physicians to educate and aid in the prevention of fish-borne zoonoses.[13]

REFERENCES

1. Chow S, Stroebel A, Lau J, et al. Mycobacterium marinum infection of the hand involving deep structures. J Hand Surg 1983;8:568–73.
2. Miller R. Fish-tank granuloma. Arch Dermatol 1969;100:780.
3. Huminer D, Pitlik, S, Block C, et al. Aquarium-borne Mycobacterium marinum skin infection. Arch Dermatol 1986;122:698–703.
4. Baily J, Stevens S, Bell W, et al. Mycobacterium marinum infection: a fishy story. JAMA 1982;247:1314.

5. Collins C, Grange J, Noble W, et al. *Mycobacterium marinum* infections in man. J Hyg Camb 1985;94:135–49.
6. Flowers D. Human infection due to *Mycobacterium marinum* after a dolphin bite. J Clin Pathol 1970;23:475–77.
7. Barrow G, Hewitt M. Skin infection with *Mycobacterium marinum* from a tropical fish tank. Br Med J 1971;2:505–6.
8. Lehane L, Rawlin G. Topically acquired bacterial zoonoses from fish: a review. Med J Aust 2000;173(5):256–9.
9. Clarridge J, Musher, Fainstein V, et al. Extraintestinal human infection caused by *Edwardsiella tarda*. J Clin Microbiol1980;11:511–4.
10. Childs J, Shope R, Fish D, et al. Emerging zoonoses. Emerging Infect Dis 1998;4(3): 453.
11. Lowry T, Smith S. Aquatic zoonses associated with food, bait, ornamental, and tropical fish. JAVMA 2007;231(6):876–80.
12. Angulo F, Glaser C, Juranek D, et al. Caring for pets of immunocompromised persons. JAVMA 1994;1:711–8.
13. Grant S, Olsen C. Preventing zoonotic diseases in immunocompromised persons: the role of physicians and veterinarians. Emerg Infect Dis 1999;5:159–63.
14. Smith A, Berry E, Skilling D, et al. In vitro isolation and characterization of a calicivirus causing a vesicular disease of the hands and feet. Clin Infect Dis 1998;26:434–9.
15. Sholtz T. Parasites in cultured and feral fish. Vet Parasitol 1999;84:317–35.
16. Hunter P, Thompson A. The zoonotic transmission of giardia and cryptosporidium. Int J Parasit 2005;35:1181–90.
17. Conrad P, Miller M, Kreuder C, et al. Transmission of toxoplasma: clues from the study of sea otters as sentinels of *Toxoplasma gondii* flow into the marine environment. Int J Parasit 2005;35:1155–68.
18. Chai J, Murrell K, Lymbery A. Fish-borne parasitic zoonoses: status and issues. Int J Parasit 2005;35:1233–54.
19. McCarthy J, Moore T. Emerging helminth zoonoses. Int J Parasit 2000;30:1351–60.
20. Macpherson C. Human behavior and the epidemiology of parasitic zoonoses. Int J Parasit 2005;35:1319–31.
21. Schwartz D. Cholangioacarcinoma associated with liver fluke infection: a preventable source of morbidity in Asian immigrants. Am J Gastroenterol 1986;81:76–9.
22. Kim K, Kim C, Lee H, et al. Biliary papillary hyperplasia with clonorchiasis resembling chlolangiocarcinoma. Am J Gastroenterol 1999;94:514–7.
23. Fries L, Williams D, Johnson S. Occurrence of *Anguillicola crassus*, an exotic parasitic swim bladder nematode of eels, in the southeastern United States. Trans Am Fisheries Soc 1996;125:794–7.
24. Barse A, Secor D. An exotic nematode parasite of the American eel. Fisheries 1999;24:6–10.
25. Sokolowski M, Dove A. Histopathological examination of wild American eels infected with *Anguillicola crassus*. J Aquatic Anim Health 2006;18:257–62.
26. Nyaoke A, Weber E, Innis C, et al. Disseminated phaeohyphomycosis in weedy seadragons (*Phyllopteryx taeniolatus*) and leafy seadragons (*Phycodurus eques*) caused by species of Exophiala, including a novel species. J Vet Diagn Invest 2009;21(1):69–79.
27. Otis EJ, Wolke RE, Blazer VS. Infection of *Exophiala salmonis* in Atlantic salmon (*Salmo salar*). J Wildl Dis 1985;21:61–4.
28. Bostock DE, Coloe PJ, Castellani A. Phaeohyphomycosis caused by *Exophiala jeanselmei* in a domestic cat. J Comp Pathol 1982;92:479–82.

29. Helms SR, McLeod CG. Systemic *Exophiala jeanselmei* infection in a cat. JAVMA 2000;217:1858–61.
30. Noga E. Post mortem techniques. In: Noga E, editor. Fish disease, diagnosis and treatment. 2nd edition. Ames (IA): Iowa State University Press: 2010. p. 63–4.
31. Kaattari IM, Rhodes MW, Kaattari SL, et al. The evolving story of *Mycobacterium tuberculosis* clade members detected in fish. J Fish Dis 2006;29:509–20.
32. Jacobs J, Stine C, Baya A, et al. A review of mycobacteriosis in marine fish. J Fish Dis 2009;32:119–30.
33. Aubry A, Chosidow O, Caumes E, et al. Sixty-three cases of Mycobacterium marinum infection. Arch Intern Med 2002;162:1746–52.
34. Jernigan J, Farr B. Incubation period and sources of exposure for cutaneous Mycobacterium marinum infection: case report and review of the literature. Clin Infect Dis 2000;31:439–43.
35. Tchornobay A, Claudy A, Perrot JL, et al. Fatal disseminated mycobacterium marinum infection. Int J Dermatol 1992;31(4):286–7.
36. Broadley S, Jenkins P, Furr J, et al. Anti-myobacterial activity of biocides. Lett Appl Microbiol 1991;13:118–22.
37. Taylor R, Falkinham J, Norton C, et al. Chlorine, chloramine, chlorine dioxide, and ozone susceptibility of Mycobacterium avium. Appl Environ Microbiol 2000;66(4):1702–5.
38. Broadley SJ, Furr JR, Jenkins PA, et al. Antimycobacterial activity of Virkon. J Hosp Infect 1993;23:189–97.
39. Mainous M, Smith S. Efficacy of common disinfectants against *Mycobacterium marinum*. J Aquatic Anim Health 2005;17:284–8.
40. Selkon J, Babb J, Morris R. Evaluation of the antimicrobial activity of a new super-oxidized water, Sterilox®, for the disinfection of endoscopes. J Hosp Infect 1999;41:59–70.
41. Babb J, Bradley C, Friase A. Glutaraldehyde-resistant *Mycobacterium chelonae* from endoscope washer disinfectors. J Appl Microbiol 1997;82(4):519–26.
42. Dantec C, Duguet J, Montiel A, et al. Chlorine disinfection of atypical mycobacteria isolated from a water distribution system. Appl Environ Microbiol 2002;68(3):1025–32.
43. Harriff M, Bermudez L, Kent M. Experimental exposure of zebrafish, *Danio rerio* (Hamilton), to *Mycobacterium marinum* and *Mycobacterium peregrinum* reveals the gastrointestinal tract as the primary route of infection: a potential model for environmental mycobacterial infection. J Fish Dis 2007;30(10):587–600.
44. Schulze-Robbecke R, Buchholtz K. Heat susceptibility of aquatic mycobacteria. Appl Environ Microbiol 1992;58(6):1869–73.
45. Agnew W, Barnes A. *Streptococcus iniae*: an aquatic pathogen of global veterinary significance and a challenging candidate for reliable vaccination. Vet Microbiol 2007;122:1–15.
46. Pier G, Madin S. *Streptococcus iniae* sp. nov., a beta-hemolytic streptococcus isolated from an Amazon freshwater dolphin, *Inia geoffrensis*. Int J Syst Bacteriol 1976;26:545–53.
47. Perera R, Johnson S, Collins M. *Streptococcus iniae* associated with mortality of tilapia nilotica × T. aurea hybrids. J Aquatic Anim Health 1994;6:335–40.
48. Shoemaker C, Klesius P, Evans J. Prevalence of *Streptococcus iniae* in tilapia, hybrid striped bass, and channel catfish on commercial fish farms in the United States. Am J Vet Res 2001;62(2):174–7.

49. Bowser P, Wooser G, Getchell R, et al. *Streptococcus iniae* infection of tilapia *Oreochromis niloticus* in a recirculation production facility. J World Aquaculture Soc 1998;29(3): 335–9.
50. Weinstein M, Litt M, Kertesz D, et al. Invasive infections due to a fish pathogen, *Streptococcus iniae*. N Engl J Med 1997;337:589–94.
51. Facklam R, Elliot J, Shewmaker L, et al. Identification and charactization of sporadic isolates of *Streptococcus iniae* isolated from humans. J Clin Microbiol 2005;43: 933–7.
52. Koh T, Kurup A, Chen J. *Streptococcus iniae* discitis in Singapore. Emerg Infect Dis 2004;10:1694–6.
53. Reidarson T. Cetacea. In: Fowler M, editor. Zoo and wild animal medicine. 5th edition. 2003. St. Louis (MO): Saunders 2003. p. 442–59.
54. Dunn L. Bacterial and mycotic diseases of cetaceans and pinnipeds. In: Dierauf L, editor. CRC handbook of marine mammal medicine: health, disease, and rehabilitation. Boca Raton (FL): CRC Press; 1990. p. 73–87.
55. Gorby G, Peacock J. *Erysipelothrix rhusiopathiae* endocarditis: microbiologic, epidemiologic, and clinical features of an occupational disease. Rev Infect Dis 1988;10(2): 317–25.
56. Klauder J, Kramor D, Nicholas L, et al. *Erysipelothrix rhusiopathiae* septicemia: diagnosis and treatment: report of fatal case of erysipeloid. JAMA 1943;122(14): 938–43.
57. Vartian C, Septimus E. Soft-tissue infection caused by *Edwardsiella tarda* and *Aeromonas hydrophila*. J Infect Dis 1990;161(4):816.
58. Noga E. Diagnoses made by bacterial culture of kidney or affected organs. In: Noga E, editor. Fish disease, diagnosis and treatment. 2nd edition. Ames (IA): Iowa State University Press; 2010. p. 185–90.
59. Khardori N, Fainstein V. Aeromonas and Plesiomonas as etiological agents. Annu Rev Microbiol 1988;42:395–419.
60. Wolf J. Aquatic animal health. In Proceedings: the second international conference on recirculating aquaculture. Roanoke (VA); 1998. p. 162–70.
61. Weise E. Spread of zoonotic agents by foods of animal origin. Dtsch Tierarztl Wochenschr 2001;108(8):344–7.
62. Austin B. *Vibrios* as causal agents of zoonoses. Vet Microbiol 2010;140:310–7.
63. Lee K, Liu P, Huang C. *Vibrio parahaemolyticus* infectious for both humans and edible mollusk abalone. Microbes Infect 2003;5(6):481–5.
64. Noga E. Post mortem techniques. In: Noga E, editor. Fish disease, diagnosis and treatment. 2nd edition. Ames (IA): Iowa State University Press; 2010. p. 192–3.
65. Janda J, Abbott S. Infections associated with the genus Edwardsiella: the role of *Edwardsiella tarda* in human disease. Clin Infect Dis 1993;17(4):742–8.
66. Slaven E, Lopez F, Hart S, et al. Myonecrosis caused by *Edwardsiella tarda*: a case report and case series of extraintestinal *E. tarda* infections. Clin Infect Dis 2001;32(10): 1430–3.
67. Wilson J, Waterer R, Wofford J, et al. Serious infections with *Edwardsiella tarda*. A case report and review of the literature. Arch Intern Med 1989;149(1):208–10.
68. Bartlett K, Trust T, Lior H. Small pet aquarium frogs as a source of Salmonella. Appl Environ Microbiol 1977;33(5):1026–9.
69. Bradley T, Angula F, Mitchell M. Public health education on *Salmonella* spp and reptiles. J Am Vet Med Assoc 2001;219(6):754–5.
70. Soto E, Hawke J, Fernandez D, et al. Francisella sp., an emerging pathogen of tilapia, *Oreochromis niloticus* in Costa Rica. J Fish Dis 2009;32(8):713–22.

71. Mauel M, Soto E, Morale M, et al. Piscirickettsiosis-like syndrome in cultured Nile Tilapia in Latin America with *Francisella* spp. as the pathogenic agent. J Aquatic Anim Health 2007;19:27–34.

72. Murrell K. Fishborne zoonotic parasites: epidemiology, detection, and elimination. In: Safety and quality issues in fish processing. Cambridge: Woodhead Publishing Ltd; 2002. p. 114–41.

73. Chen H. Seafood microorganisms and seafood safety. J Food Drug Analy 1995;3: 133–44.

Zoonotic Diseases Associated with Reptiles and Amphibians: An Update

Mark A. Mitchell, DVM, MS, PhD, Dip. ECZM (Herpetology)

KEYWORDS

• Reptiles • Amphibians • Bacteria • Parasites • Viruses
• Fungi

Reptiles and amphibians are popular pets in the United States and Europe. The most recent American Veterinary Medical Association market research statistics for US pet ownership (2007) reported that there has been an increase in the number of households maintaining reptiles, with more than 600,000 new households reporting reptile pet ownership since the 2001 market statistics were published. Although this increase in pet reptile ownership is positive for veterinarians and herpetoculturists interested in the captive care and management of these animals, it has also caused increased concerns among public health officials because of the zoonotic potential associated with these animals. Encounters with reptiles and amphibians are also on the rise in the laboratory setting (eg, African clawed frogs, *Xenopus laevis*) and with wild animals (eg, wildlife rehabilitation facilities); in both of these practices, there is also an increased likelihood for exposure to zoonotic pathogens. Veterinarians working with reptiles and amphibians can serve as important educators to clients, laboratory personnel, and the public at large when they encounter these animals. It is important that veterinarians remain current with the literature as it relates to emerging and reemerging zoonotic diseases attributed to reptiles and amphibians so that they can protect themselves, their staff, and their clients from potential problems.

Although *Salmonella* spp. has received the greatest amount of attention regarding zoonoses associated with reptiles and amphibians, there are other emerging pathogens that should also be considered (eg, *Mycobacteria* spp, West Nile virus [WNV]). Limiting our concerns and focusing on a single pathogen group (eg, *Salmonella* in reptiles) can be detrimental to our ability to diagnose and manage these pathogens. The purpose of this review article was to provide some insight into the background of common and emerging zoonotic pathogens associated with reptiles and amphibians.

Department of Veterinary Clinical Medicine, University of Illinois, College of Veterinary Medicine, 1008 West Hazelwood Drive, Urbana, IL 61820, USA
E-mail address: mmitch@illinois.edu

Vet Clin Exot Anim 14 (2011) 439–456
doi:10.1016/j.cvex.2011.05.005
1094-9194/11/$ – see front matter © 2011 Elsevier Inc. All rights reserved.

By making veterinarians aware of these disease organisms, it increases the likelihood that diagnostic workups will account for these pathogens and that clients will be informed as to the potential risks associated with these disease agents.

BACTERIA

Bacteria are the group that receives the most attention as potential zoonotic pathogens from reptiles and amphibians. Although parasites, viruses, and fungi from reptiles can also potentially be zoonotic, they are rare by comparison. The primary reasons that bacteria are more successful as zoonotic pathogens is that they have logarithmic growth rates, are tolerant of a wide variety of environmental temperatures and humidities, and can colonize a variety of surfaces in the artificial environments created by humans. Taking these factors into account is important when trying to eliminate and/or suppress these potential pathogens.[1-4]

Any bacteria harbored in a reptile or amphibian (or their environment) could cause a zoonotic infection if the human in contact with the animal has a compromised immune system. It is for this reason that strict hygiene should always be practiced. The bacteria outlined in this article represent those that are most commonly associated with reptiles and amphibians and is not meant to be an all-inclusive list.

Salmonella

Salmonella are Gram-negative, usually motile, facultative anaerobes that conform to the definition of the family Enterobacteriaceae. These bacteria have a cosmopolitan distribution.[5] There are currently more than 2400 recognized serotypes of *Salmonella*, and many public health officials consider all serotypes to be pathogenic.[6] However, it is important to recognize that these organisms are not pathogenic under all conditions. In reptiles and amphibians, *Salmonella* is considered a component of their indigenous microflora[7]; most reptiles and amphibians that are culture positive show no signs of clinical disease. This type of information is frequently used by public health officials as a basis for defending current legislation against the sale of chelonians less than 10.2 cm^3 and creating local responses against pet ownership of reptiles; however, similar reports of *Salmonella* isolation from clinically normal dogs,[8,9] cats,[10,11] and rodents[12] are available. This discrepancy can lead to a lack of awareness of the risk(s) associated with these mammalian pets, and it is important for veterinarians to reinforce the practice of handwashing and proper disinfection when working with any pet. It is certainly prudent to be careful when working with reptiles, but this author follows the same precautions when working with any animal.

In the past 15 years, the classification of *Salmonella* has been reorganized. The current classification of the genus *Salmonella* includes 2 species, *S enterica* and *S bongori*; *S enterica* is the species of concern as it relates to reptiles and amphibians. There are 6 subspecies of *S enterica*, including *enterica* (subspecies I), *salamae* (subspecies II), *arizonae* (subspecies III), *diarizonae* (subspecies IIIb), *houtenae* (subspecies IV), and *indica* (subspecies V).[13] Subspecies I is routinely isolated from humans, whereas the other subspecies are frequently isolated from poikilotherms and the environment. *Salmonella* are serotyped according to their O (heat stable somatic) antigen, Vi (heat labile capsular) antigen, and H (flagellar) antigen. Serotyping is important when characterizing the different organisms, because some are currently only classified based on these antigens. The use of serotyping can be especially useful in epidemiologic investigations attempting to determine the source of infection in human cases. While serotyping remains an important method for characterizing *Salmonella* in reptile-associated salmonellosis cases, other methods are also being used including phage typing, evaluating antibiotic resistance patterns, plasmid profiles, and biotyping.

Salmonella and reptiles: a brief history

The relationship between reptiles and *Salmonella* is not recent. *Salmonella* was first isolated from a lizard (*Heloderma suspectum*) in 1944,[14] although an earlier unconfirmed report of an organism consistent with the biochemical attributes of *Salmonella* was isolated from 3 dead, wild-caught Gila monsters in 1939.[15] *Salmonella* was also isolated from a snake for the first time around the same time. A gopher snake (*Pituophis catenifer deserticola*) killed on a turkey farm for eating turkey poults was found to harbor 3 different serotypes; it was the first report of multiple serotypes being isolated from the same reptile.[16] The first report of a *Salmonella* being isolated from a chelonian involved *Salmonella* Newport, which was isolated from the liver, spleen, lungs, and intestine of a Galapagos tortoise (*Geochelone giganteas*) at necropsy.[14] These initial reports showed that *Salmonella* could be isolated from both wild and captive animals.

Turtle-associated salmonellosis in humans

Reptile-associated salmonellosis was being reported in humans soon after *Salmonella* was isolated from reptiles. The first case of turtle-associated salmonellosis in humans was reported in 1943,[17] and the frequency of cases increased over the next 20 years.[18] However, it was not until 1963 that the first case of turtle-associated salmonellosis in a child was reported.[19] *Salmonella* Hartford was recovered from a 7-month-old infant with diarrhea, vomiting, and fever. An investigation of the infant's environment resulted in the isolation of the same serotype from the family's pet turtle.

The increased frequency of turtle-associated salmonellosis in children was of concern to both state and federal health officials. In an attempt to estimate the magnitude of turtle-associated salmonellosis in the United States, retrospective surveys of laboratory-confirmed cases were reviewed to determine frequency of turtle ownership with data from various state and county health agencies, including Utah, Atlanta, Georgia, Santa Clara County, California, and Seattle, Washington.[20] A retrospective, case-control study was also conducted on cases reported in Connecticut. Twenty-four percent of the salmonellosis cases in Connecticut were associated with an exposure to a turtle, compared with 2% of the controls. The findings in the other parts of the country varied, with salmonellosis cases in Santa Clara, California, reporting an association with turtles in 18% of the cases, 15.6% in Utah, 11.6% in Seattle, and 10.9% in Atlanta.[20] This information was then combined with previous turtle-associated salmonellosis reports in an uncontrolled study in Minnesota (turtle exposure: 25%)[19] and a controlled study in New Jersey (turtle exposure cases, 22.6%; controls, 5.7%).[21] An estimate of the number of turtle-associated salmonellosis cases in the United States was then developed. The proportion of juvenile salmonellosis cases associated with exposure to turtles was averaged among the 7 sites to yield a mean of 18.2%. This average was then applied to the estimated number of salmonellosis cases in the United States (2,000,000), assuming that turtles were present in 4.2% of US households. The estimate of the total number of households at risk was determined by a calculation derived from the number of turtles sold in a given year (in 1971, 15,000,000) and the number of households in the United States (in 1971, 60,000,000). The estimate of 4.2% corresponds with the number of households that maintained a turtle in the Connecticut and New Jersey studies.[20] Based on these reference parameters, approximately 14% (280,000) of the salmonellosis cases in the United States in 1971 were turtle associated.

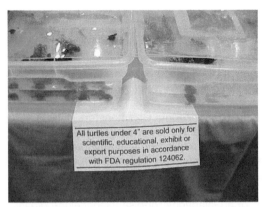

Fig. 1. Although the US FDA instituted a regulation in 1975 restricting the sale of turtles less than 10.2 cm, many herpetoculturists sell the turtles by promoting the "educational" value of the turtles. Although not the intent of the regulation, there is limited enforcement.

To stem the disease issues being reported in children, the US Food and Drug Administration (FDA) enacted a regulation in 1975 that restricted the interstate shipment of all turtle eggs and live turtles with a carapace length of less than 10.2 cm (**Fig. 1**). The decision to restrict the sale of turtles with a carapace length of less than 10.2 cm was based on the assumption that animals larger than that would be less desirable to young children. Enforcement of this policy resulted in a 77% reduction in the incidence of cases in those states without indigenous production of turtles.[22] However, it is important to consider that the actual number of cases monitored in the reduction was less than 300.

Since the enforcement of the 1975 FDA regulation, there has been an extended period where turtle-associated salmonellosis outbreaks have been limited to sporadic local events; however, since 2006, there have been 3 multistate outbreaks documented in the United States.[23] Much of this seems to be related to poor decision making by the individuals purchasing the animals, such as spontaneous purchases, new owners being unprepared for caring for the animals, and poor hygiene and husbandry. Although these seem to be grounds for public health officials to take aggressive tones with those breeding and selling reptiles, it is important to recognize that similar outbreaks are commonly reported with foods, food products, pet products, and captive rodents without a similar response by the government.

Attempts to reduce or eliminate *Salmonella* in turtles with antimicrobials were initiated after the FDA regulation was implemented in 1975. Treatment of hatchlings with oxytetracycline in their tank water for up to 14 days alleviated shedding in treated turtles, but did not affect systemic infection.[24] Treatment of the freshly laid eggs with oxytetracycline or chloramphenicol with a temperature differential egg dip method was successful at eliminating *Salmonella* in eggs less than 1 day old, but did not clear eggs greater than 2 days old.[24] Large-scale experimentation on commercial turtle farms with surface decontamination and pressure or temperature differential treatment of eggs with gentamicin dip solutions for eggs greater than 2 days old, followed by hatching the eggs on *Salmonella*-free bedding, substantially reduced *Salmonella* infections and shedding rates in hatchling turtles.[25] Forty percent of the eggs not treated with the gentamicin were found to harbor *Salmonella*, whereas only 0.15% of the treated eggs were positive. Legislative implementation of this concurrent method of surface decontamination and gentamicin treatment by the Louisiana Department of Agriculture in 1985 was hailed as victory by turtle farmers. Unfortunately, use of gentamicin and the other antimicrobials has led to an even greater concern owing to the development and persistence of antimicrobial-resistant strains of *Salmonella*.[26,27]

Because of the concerns related to antimicrobial resistance, more recent attempts to suppress and/or eliminate *Salmonella* in turtles or their environment have used non-antibiotic compounds.[1–4] Polyhexamethylene biguanide has been used by the author successfully to significantly reduce the prevalence/incidence of *Salmonella* in the eggshell, hatchling, aquatic habitat, and transport water of red-eared slider turtles (*Trachemys scripta elegans*).[1–3] Although not perfect, these findings mimic those reported by the poultry industry, where complete elimination of the pathogen is not possible, but suppression and reduction of the prevalence is. The author expects that reptile caretakers will need to use these types of antimicrobials, in addition to proper husbandry (eg, appropriate environmental temperature, *Salmonella*-free diet), to minimize stress and the potential shedding of *Salmonella* in the captive environment of reptiles and amphibians.

Reptile-associated salmonellosis in humans

Although the 1975 US FDA regulation did reduce the number of turtle associated salmonellosis cases, it has had no effect on the number of non-chelonian reptile associated salmonellosis cases. According to the US Centers for Disease Control and Prevention (CDC), the incidence of reptile-associated salmonellosis cases in humans has increased dramatically over the past several decades.[28] In 1996, the CDC estimated that reptiles accounted for 3% to 5% of the 2 to 6 million cases of human salmonellosis in the United States.[29] In most documented reptile-associated cases of salmonellosis, the strain of *Salmonella* isolated from the patient was common to the pet reptile, suggesting the source of infection.[30] The increased incidence of reptile-associated salmonellosis has been associated with the increased popularity of these animals as pets during the past 2 decades. From 1989 to 1993, imports increased 82%, from 1.1 million to 2.1 million animals. Green iguanas accounted for the greatest proportion, with imports increasing by 431% from 143,000 to 760,000. More recent data suggest that the number of reptiles being imported into the United States increased by 20% (2.5 million reptiles),[31] with a 2009 National Pet Owner's Survey reporting 13.6 million pet reptiles in the United States.

Atypical serotypes of *Salmonella* have been anecdotally associated with reptile ownership. Cieslak and colleagues[32] defined and described the epidemiology of reptile-associated serotypes (RAS) in the United States. RAS of *Salmonella* were defined as those in which reptilian sources composed the majority of the reports of non-human isolates reported to the CDC between 1981 and 1990. Human isolates of RAS reported to the CDC between 1970 and 1992 were analyzed and incidence rates calculated by age, gender, state, and year. A 1991 American Veterinary Medical Association Survey was used to compare reptile ownership with rates of RAS isolation by state. The annual incidence of RAS increased from $2.4/10^7$ persons per year in 1970 to $8.4/10^7$ persons per year in 1992. This rise in cases represents a total of 150 new cases per year based on United State population estimates. Although pet reptile ownership has been reported to be increasing (7.3 million reptiles; CDC, 1995; 13.6 million pet reptiles in the United States in 2009, National Pet Owner's Survey), estimates of annual turtle sales in 1971 (15,000,000 turtles)[20] far exceed these more recent estimates of pet animals. The increased incidence of RAS may be associated with improved clinical diagnostic techniques, a higher carriage rate in squamates (non-chelonian reptiles), or the duration of exposure to the pet. The average life span of an aquatic turtle in captivity in 1971 was estimated to be less than 2 months,[20] whereas the average longevity of squamates in captivity in 2011 (as well as chelonians >10.2 cm) is likely far greater than 2 months because of improved husbandry techniques.

A matched case-control study was performed with the 1993 New York state *Salmonella* surveillance database to further assess the epidemiology of reptile-associated salmonellosis.[33] Case selection included those individuals with *Salmonella* serotypes common to reptiles or characterized in reports of reptile-associated salmonellosis. RAS of *Salmonella* were defined as those which reptilian sources composed the majority of the reports of non-human isolates reported to the CDC between 1981 and 1990.[32] The RAS included 35 serotypes of *Salmonella* type I; all serotypes in II, III, and IV; and 10 other serotypes linked to human RAS cases. Each case was matched by age (<5 years of age within 2 years; 5–21 years of age within 3 years; and >21 years of age within 10 years) and date of diagnosis (within 30 days) to 1 or 2 controls (*Shigella* cases), reported to the NY Department of Health in the same year. Telephone surveys were conducted on all available cases and controls to acquire data on symptoms, hospitalization, pet ownership, exposure to reptiles, and dietary habits. Of the 1362 *Salmonella* serotypes, 42 (3%) were considered RAS. Of these 42 cases, 24 (57%) were interviewed. Twelve (50%) of the cases reported reptile ownership, as compared with only 2 of the 28 controls (matched odds ratio [OR], 6.6; 95% confidence interval [CI], 1.4–31.0). Ten of the cases had specific contact with iguanas, whereas none of the controls reported having contact with an iguana. It has been estimated that approximately 5% of all salmonellosis cases are reported.[34] Using this estimate, there would have been in excess of 700 RAS cases in New York state during 1993. The findings suggest that reptile-associated salmonellosis is more than an incidental occurrence.

Outbreaks of RAS are rare in zoologic institutions, despite the fact that 95% of the 174 zoos and aquariums in North America affiliated with the American Zoo and Aquarium Association exhibit reptiles.[35] In January 1996, *Salmonella enteritidis* was isolated from the feces of several children living in Jefferson County, Colorado.[36] The only common link among these patients was that they had visited an exhibit of Komodo dragons held over a 9-day period at the Denver Zoological Gardens. An epidemiologic investigation (matched case-control study) was conducted to assess the extent of the outbreak. A confirmed case was defined as an individual that had gastrointestinal disease and an isolate of *S enteritidis* from a fecal sample during the specified time period (January 11–21, 1996). A suspect case was one that attended the exhibit during the specified time period and experienced gastrointestinal disease. A secondary case was defined as an individual classified as a case or suspect, but who became ill subsequent to a case-patient in the household. Controls were selected from the list of zoo patrons who participated in a promotional event that took place during the exhibit. Cases and controls were matched according to 1 of 9 age groups and the day they attended the exhibit. A telephone interview was performed to identify cases and controls and to elicit demographic data, medical history, exposure, and activity at the zoo. Culture samples were also collected from the Komodo dragons, their environment, food source (rats), and the zoo keepers working with these animals.

There were 39 culture-confirmed cases and 26 suspect cases. Forty-eight case individuals, comprising 33 culture-confirmed and 15 suspects, were the first to become ill in their households. The median age of the patients was 7 years (range, 3 months–48 years); 53 (82%) were under 13 years old and 34 (55%) were male. The median time until the onset of disease was 3.5 days. *S enteritidis* was isolated from only 1 of the 4 Komodo dragons at the exhibit. The phage type 8 isolate was common to the case patients. The same organism was also isolated on 3 occasions from the barrier wall that separated the animals and the visitors. Visitors were allowed to rest their hands and elbows on the barrier surface, which was also accessible to the animals. Direct contact with the reptiles was limited, with only 2 controls touching an animal. Twenty-six cases were matched to 49 controls for the case-control study. There was a significant risk associated with touching the barrier that housed the dragons (OR, 4.0; 95% CI, 1.2–13.9). Handwashing after visiting the exhibit or prior to the next meal was found to be protective (OR, 0.1; 95% CI, 0.02–0.50). There was no difference between the groups when comparing the risk of eating food purchased at zoo concessions or touching a reptile skin on display at the exhibit. This report described the first known outbreak of reptile-associated salmonellosis at a zoologic park and reinforces that *Salmonella* can be transmitted from reptiles to humans without direct contact.

In addition to these case-control studies, case reports continue to be published acknowledging non-chelonian reptiles as sources of *Salmonella* in humans. Since 2000, there have been cases attributed to bearded dragons (*Pogona vitticeps*),[37,38] boa constrictors (*Boa constrictor*),[39] and green iguanas (*Iguana iguana*).[39] The findings in bearded dragons are very interesting, because these animals are now being captive raised in large numbers (**Fig. 2**). Unlike green iguanas and boas, which can become quite large, bearded dragons are a small to moderately sized animal. This smaller size is one of the reasons these animals are popular pets, especially around children. The examples in the literature of bearded dragon-associated salmonellosis should remind veterinarians of the risk these animals may pose to their caretakers, especially younger children, who may be less likely to practice appropriate disinfection after handling their pet or while cleaning and feeding it.

The Association of Reptilian and Amphibian Veterinarians has continued to update and publish guidelines for minimizing the potential for reptile-associated salmonellosis. The most recent guidelines were published in 2009.[40] Separate information is available to share with veterinary personnel and clients. Veterinarians should consider posting this information in their veterinary hospitals to remind themselves and their

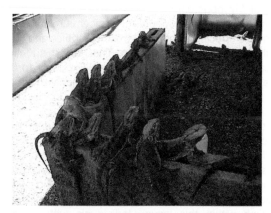

Fig. 2. It should not be unexpected that bearded dragons have been identified as a source of reptile-associated salmonellosis. These animals are typically raised in large numbers under high densities, which is a perfect environment for disseminating enteric bacteria such as *Salmonella*.

staff of the risks associated with pet reptile ownership. Veterinarians should also consider providing a copy of the document to their clients to reinforce to them the best practices for minimizing the potential for problems.

Amphibian-associated salmonellosis

Although much of the focus on *Salmonella* over the past 60 years has been directed toward reptiles, recent reports confirm that amphibians are also an important group of concern. In July 2009, the Utah Department of Health reported 5 cases of *Salmonella* Typhimurium, indistinguishable by pulsed-field gel electrophoresis, that had occurred starting in April of that year.[41] Over the course of 2009, a total of 85 patients from 31 states were identified as having the same pathogen (based on pulsed-field gel electrophoresis). A case-control study conducted during the year revealed a strong association between the human infections and exposure to African dwarf frogs (*Hymenochirus* sp; matched OR, 24.4; 95% CI, 4.0–infinity). Follow-up testing in several of the case patient's homes yielded the outbreak organism from samples of water, substrate, filters, tanks, and a dead frog. The pathogen was traced back to a breeder's facility in California. This example should not be surprising, because it is high-density breeding that typically results in the dissemination of *Salmonella*. This case should reinforce to veterinarians the potential risk associated with amphibians as potential carriers of *Salmonella*, and the same recommendations given for minimizing exposure in reptiles should be applied to amphibians too.

Reptile food sources of Salmonella

Frozen rodents intended as food for reptiles have recently been found to serve as a potential zoonotic source of *S* Typhimurium.[42] These cases are especially interesting because the reptiles consuming the mice or rats may be blamed for the human exposure, but it is the rodents that serve as the primary source of the pathogen. All vertebrates seem to be susceptible to being colonized by *Salmonella* and should be handled using best practices to minimize the potential dissemination of any potential zoonotic agents.

Mycobacteriosis

Mycobacteriosis is an important disease in humans. Whereas humans have their own particular species of *Mycobacterium* (*M tuberculosis*), there are also a number of zoonotic species from this genus. Most of the concerns related to this organism are associated with aquatic species, although terrestrial reptiles and amphibians can also serve as potential sources of this pathogen. The reason aquatic species pose a greater risk is because of the aquatic environment. Exposure to the organism does not have to come through direct contact with the animal, but can occur with the environment itself. Mycobacteria can lie dormant in these environments and exposure can occur when exchanging water, wiping down the insides of an aquarium, manipulating the substrate, or cleaning filters. Fish handler's disease is a generic name used to describe the lesions associated with the mycobacteria (*M fortuitum* and *M marinum*) infections attributed to aquarium and aquaculture species of fish. These organisms can also be found in captive aquatic reptile and amphibian aquariums. While the lesions are typically mild (eg, erythematous skin lesions), more severe cases can result in osteomyelitis and sepsis (see **Fig. 1** in Boylan's article on Zoonoses Associated with Fish within this issue). Individuals with compromised immune systems should not serve as the caretaker for aquatic habitats that hold vertebrates, because these environments can become loaded with potentially opportunistic zoonotic pathogens.

Three recent cases of mycobacteriosis in captive frogs reinforce the potential risk associated with these animals. *M chelonae* is a potential human pathogen. This organism is typically associated with fish and reptiles, but has also been identified in African clawed frogs.[43] Affected frogs had clinical signs that were consistent with mycobacteriosis in fish, including weight loss and cutaneous lesions. Confirmation of the pathogen was done using polymerase chain reaction (PCR) testing. *M gordonae*, another potential human pathogen, was also recently identified in a group of African clawed frogs.[44] The pathogen caused cutaneous nodular lesions in the frogs. These types of lesions are common in these frogs and are often attributed to trauma from conspecifics and Gram-negative infections. In some cases, the mycobacteriosis may be masked by other pathogens, as occurred in a recent case associated with a wild *Xenopus laevis* housed in a laboratory setting.[45] This frog also had concurrent *Aeromonas hydrophila* and *Batrachochytrium dendrobatidis* infections. This example is important because cases of mycobacteriosis in vertebrates typically only become evident when the host becomes stressed, increasing the potential for shedding the organism. The risk of exposure to this pathogen can be minimized by limiting the stresses associated with captivity, such as regulating animal density and optimizing water quality and nutrition.

Veterinarians working with amphibians or reptiles displaying signs consistent with chronic wasting (eg, low body condition score) or non-healing skin lesions should consider mycobacteriosis in their differential. This is important because a pathologist may need to use special stains (eg, acid-fast) or diagnostic tests (eg, PCR testing) to confirm the presence of the *Mycobacteria* sp. To minimize the risk of zoonotic infection with this organism, clients should be educated to the importance of wearing gloves when working with animals with open sores, or when the caretaker has open sores, and handwashing immediately after working in an aquatic environment.

Escherichia coli

E coli is a Gram-negative bacteria from the family Enterobacteriaceae. This organism is considered indigenous microflora in a variety of vertebrates, including humans. The pathogenicity of this organism is tied to the toxins it produces. One of the most pathogenic is the shiga-toxin producing form. *E coli* 0157 is a serotype that has been associated with severe disease in humans. Children and immunocompromised individuals tend to develop the most severe side effects, including hemolytic uremic syndrome and thrombocytopenic purpura.[46] Humans are typically exposed to this pathogen through food or contact with production animals, and ruminants are considered the natural reservoir.[47] Recent research has shown that amphibians may also play a role in the epidemiology of this pathogen. Gray and colleagues[48] were able to orally inoculate American bullfrog (*Rana catesbeiana*) metamorphs with *E coli* 0157:H7 and isolate the organism from these animals 14 days postinoculation. Because this species is native in the United States, there are concerns that it could serve as a spillover reservoir for the pathogen in the environment. These findings also suggest that these animals could serve as a source of infection to humans that maintain these animals in captivity.

Whereas the previous study found it was possible to experimentally infect amphibians with *E coli* 0157, a recent study from Italy found that frogs can be naturally infected as well.[49] Cloacal samples were collected from 60 captive frogs and their environments and evaluated for the presence of the pathogen. Two (3.3%) of the frogs were *E coli* 0157 positive. The species of frogs found to be positive, the red-eyed tree frog (*Agalychnis callidryas*) and firebelly toad (*Bombina orientalis*), are commonly kept as pets in the United States and Europe. Whereas the prevalence of

E coli 0157 was low, it is important to note that the samples were collected ante-mortem from the cloaca. This bacteria, like *Salmonella* spp, can be transiently shed so the study likely underestimated the true prevalence. Although humans typically encounter this bacterium through contaminated food, it is also possible to obtain it from close contact with live animals (eg, petting zoos).[47] Veterinarians should educate their clients to the zoonotic potential of amphibians (more specifically anurans) regarding this pathogen. Routine disinfection and handwashing should minimize the risk for exposure. To date, there have been no studies evaluating the role of reptiles in the epidemiology of *E coli* 0157.

Vancomycin-Resistant Enterococci

Multidrug-resistant bacteria are a major concern to public health officials. Of those that are followed, vancomycin-resistant enterococci are of special concern. In humans, these bacteria have been associated with a high annual mortality rate and are considered 1 of the top 3 nosocomial infections associated with hospitals.[50] Although the risk of disease within hospitals and in domestic species has been documented, there has been little research evaluating the roles of herpetofauna in the epidemiology of vancomycin-resistant enterococci. Recently, a study evaluating wild-caught wood frogs (*Rana sylvatica*) from Michigan found that amphibians can harbor organisms with these antibiotic resistance patterns.[51] *Enterococcus faecium* isolated from fecal samples of the wood frogs were found to carry similar resistance genes to those found in human isolates. The findings from the study reinforce the importance of amphibians as sentinels for disease and the general health and well-being of an ecosystem. Because wild-caught frogs are captured and sold for the pet trade, these results should also remind veterinarians of the zoonotic potential amphibians may serve when brought into captivity.

Chlamydia (Chlamydophila)

Chlamydia (*Chlamydophila*) is an important pathogen in humans. This obligate intracellular bacterium has been associated with a range of clinical presentations in humans, including fever, upper respiratory tract disease, lower respiratory tract disease, granulomatous disease, sepsis, and death. *Chlamydia pneumoniae* has historically been considered an obligate pathogen of humans. However, recent research has shown that this pathogen likely originated from animals, including reptiles and amphibians.[52,53] Mitchell and associates[52] evaluated 2 distinct lineages of *C pneumoniae*. One of the lineages includes pathogens currently found in humans across North America, the Middle East, and Asia. Based on molecular genetics, the authors suggested that this genotype originated from a reptile or amphibian lineage. Two Australian genotypes were also evaluated and they, too, seem to have an animal origin, amphibian and marsupial lines. The studies suggest that *C pneumoniae* was likely zoonotic, but over time adapted to humans through gene decay. This is an important consideration today because we are altering the environment of pathogens. Reptiles and amphibians are imported in large numbers from across the globe. Many of the pathogens that these animals harbor have likely never encountered humans before. It is possible that the current behaviors we practice (eg, pet ownership) will introduce and result in the development of new zoonotic pathogens and potential human diseases in the future. Because of these risks, it is important for veterinarians to set the standard for educating their clients about the potential risks associated with pet reptile and amphibian ownership.

Although it seems that reports of *Chlamydia* spp are recent in reptiles and amphibians, it is more likely we have only recently had the diagnostic capacity to look for this organism in these species. Recent examples show that this organism can be found in both terrestrial and aquatic reptiles and amphibians. To date, there are no documented zoonotic cases, although it is possible that some have occurred and have not been reported. Because *Chlamydia* spp have been isolated from reptiles and amphibians, it should be presumed that they can serve as hosts for the pathogen and that humans working with these animals should practice strict hygiene and sanitation to minimize the potential for being exposed to this pathogen. The following represent some recent reports of *Chlamydia* in reptiles and amphibians and should serve to remind veterinarians of the potential risks of exposure to this pathogen:

Intracytoplasmic inclusions that were *Chlamydia*-like were identified in circulating monocytes of wild flap necked chameleons (*Chamaelo dilepis*; n = 3) from Tanzania.[54] Similar inclusions were found in the spleen and liver of one of the lizards after it was euthanized. Electron microscopy and histopathology suggested the lesions were consistent with chlamydial organisms. This case was reported before more advanced testing (eg, PCR) was commercially available to confirm a chlamydial infection.

A mortality event in captive 4- to 5-year-old green sea turtles at an aquaculture facility was associated with chlamydial infection.[55] Necropsy findings from a subset of dead animals were consistent with chlamydial infection: necrotizing myocarditis, splenitis, hepatic changes, and interstitial pneumonia. Special stains and electron microscopy were used to confirm the presence of chlamydial organisms.

A mortality event in another aquaculture system, this time farm-raised Nile crocodiles (*Crocodylus niloticus*), was also associated with chlamydial infection.[56] Necropsies performed on animals that died acutely revealed edema, hepatitis, and inclusions. The outbreak was presumed to be associated with C *psittaci*. An outbreak of chlamydiosis was also reported in Indopacific crocodiles (*Crocodylus porosus*).[57] The hatchling and juvenile animals were found to have hepatitis at necropsy. In the second case, wild-caught animals brought into the aquaculture facility were considered to be the point source of the infection. These mortality events are a good reminder of the potential for rapid dissemination of highly pathogenic organisms in systems where reptiles are housed in high densities.

A collection of emerald tree boas (*Corralus caninus*) composed of both wild-caught and captive-bred animals experienced a large mortality event.[58] Necropsies of the snakes revealed granulomas that were immunoperoxidase and lipopolysaccharide antigen positive for *Chlamydia*. Follow-up work using TaqMan PCR from frozen samples from the snakes revealed that C *pneumoniae* was the cause of disease.[59] Whereas the presence of the organism in the snakes does not confirm that they can serve as a source of infection for humans, precautions should be taken when working with *Chlamydia*-positive collections.

There are several reports of *Chlamydia* (*Chlamydophila*) infections in anurans, with most cases being associated with *Xenopus* spp. One of the first reports of infection was attributed to C *psittaci* in X *laevis*.[60] Affected animals were found to have pyogranulomatous disease. Further diagnostics, including histopathology, electron microscopy, and cell culture, were used to confirm the chlamydial infection. Reed and co-workers[61] reported a mortality event in imported X *tropicalis*, in which 90% of the animals being imported died from an epizootic of C *pneumoniae*. This case, like the previous example for emerald tree boas, reinforces the importance of follow-through with confirming an epizootic and the need to take special precautions with *Chlamydia*-positive collections.

PARASITES

Reptiles and amphibians can play different roles in the dissemination of parasites. The greatest risk for zoonoses would be expected when the reptile or amphibian serves as the definitive host, where it can shed the organism into its environment and potentially expose human caretakers. When reptiles or amphibians serve as an intermediate host, the risk is lower, except for cases where the reptile is consumed. In many parts of the world, reptiles and amphibians are an important source of dietary protein; in these cases, the risk of exposure to zoonotic parasites when the reptile or amphibian serves as an intermediate host should also be considered. Because the intent of this article is to focus on captive and pet animals, the summary of potential parasitic zoonoses focuses on this group.

Pentastomes are worm-like endoparasites. These organisms have been assigned to their own phylum, *Pentastomida*, although they share common characteristics with annelids and arthropods. The adult stages of these parasites are typically found in the respiratory tract of reptiles. The greatest concern for zoonoses with these parasites is related to consumption and handling of wild animals.[62] The reason to discuss them here is because wild-caught snakes can harbor these parasites and bring them into the captive environment. Humans can potentially be exposed when handling contaminated environmental products (eg, substrate or water) or fecal material/sputum. The risk of zoonoses can be minimized by practicing strict hygiene and sanitation. All wild-caught reptiles should be screened for endo- and ectoparasites to minimize the potential for introducing these organisms into the captive environment. In the case of pentastomes, fecal and sputum samples could be collected and screened. The author recommends screening wild reptiles over several months to increase the likelihood of identifying parasites that are being transiently shed.

Cryptosporidiosis is a plague among reptile collections. This parasite, a member of the apicomplexans, is highly contagious, difficult to treat, and associated with high morbidity and mortality in reptile collections. *Cryptosporidium serpentis* is the parasite associated with snakes. It can cause a severe gastritis that leads to an animal having an inability to "hold down food." Over time, these animals tend to lose body condition and become dehydrated. Initial attempts to determine whether *C serpentis* could cross-infect other vertebrates (ducklings) were unsuccessful; therefore, it is assumed that this parasite is group (snake) specific.[63] *C saurophilum* is the parasite typically associated with lizards. It has been associated with high mortality rates in leopard geckos (*Eublepharis macularius*). More recently, cryptosporidiosis has been reported in chelonians.[64,65] As with the lizards and snakes, pathology was identified in the gastrointestinal tract of the tortoises (gastric and intestinal).[64] Although there is work left to be done in characterizing these organisms, in at least 1 report the organism isolated from tortoises (*Testudo graeca*, *T hermanni*, *T marginata*) has been associated with zoonoses (*Cryptosporidium pestis* [*Cryptosporidium parvum* 'bovine genotype']; **Fig. 3**).[65] Because these organisms are shed freely into the environment, it is important that clients be educated regarding the importance of following strict hygiene and sanitation protocols to minimize the potential for being exposed to these or other potentially zoonotic agents.

Ticks and mites are examples of arthropods that parasitize reptiles. Ticks are commonly found on recently imported reptiles, although captive animals sharing space with wild-caught animals may also be parasitized. Although these organisms rarely cause overt disease in reptiles, the possibility exists that they can serve as vectors for disease. Although some of these diseases may only affect reptiles, it is

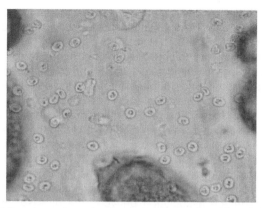

Fig. 3. *Cryptosporidium* is an important parasite in reptiles. Historically, the species of *Cryptosporidium* found in reptiles have not been considered zoonotic, although a recent report suggests that they may harbor species that have been identified as zoonotic.

possible that some can also affect humans. The best way to minimize the risk of zoonoses associated with ticks is to remove them at the time of examination.

Snake mites (*Ophionyssus natricis*) are a common ectoparasite of captive snakes. Unlike ticks, these ectoparasites can establish high densities within a reptile enclosure, leading to severe disease in some animals (eg, young snakes). These organisms can also serve as vectors for disease, and therefore should be eliminated. Although not considered a major zoonotic concern, snake mites can aggravate humans, as fleas do, and cause a mild dermatitis **(Fig. 4)**.[66]

VIRUSES

It should be no surprise to veterinarians who work with reptiles that these animals are not commonly associated with viruses that are zoonotic, because we only recently have developed the diagnostic capability of identifying viruses in reptiles.

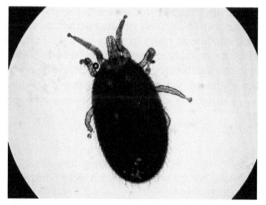

Fig. 4. Snake mites, like fleas, can overtake an environment. Although not commonly a problem in humans, examples of localized mite infestation on susceptible humans have been reported.

As our capacity grows for characterizing viruses in reptiles, we may see an increased number of viruses being associated with zoonotic infections. To date, 1 virus fits this example: WNV.

WNV is a flavivirus that was first reported in the United States in 1999. Although much of the epidemiology of this disease was found to be dependent on birds, at least 1 reptile was also found to play a role in its epidemiology.[67] Infected American alligators (*Alligator mississipiensis*) have been found to become viremic and shed WNV in their feces. The reason this disease became important in the alligator industry is because it was associated with lymphoplasmacytic syndrome of alligators, or "Pix" as it is called by alligator ranchers. This disease was first reported in Louisiana in 2001, the same time WNV was first documented in the state. The lesions that are found in the skin can be significant, reducing the value of the leather or causing it to be rejected outright. Antibody testing and PCR have been used to confirm the association between the disease and the histologic findings. At least 2 human WNV cases have been reported in individuals working on alligator farms. In both cases, WNV was also reported in alligators on the farm. Because the alligators can shed the virus, and the environment itself is predisposed to vectors that carry the virus, veterinarians and personnel on the farms should take special precautions (eg, wear gloves, mosquito control) when working on site.

FUNGI

Although there are no reports of zoonotic fungi associated with reptiles, it is important to recognize that these animals or their environment can serve as reservoirs for potentially pathogenic/opportunistic fungi. Human caretakers of reptiles that have compromised immune systems may be more susceptible to infections. Individuals that are at increased risk for acquiring zoonotic or nosocomial infections should not handle or care for reptiles.

SUMMARY

Reptiles have long been implicated as important sources of zoonotic pathogens (eg, *Salmonella*). Although at one level this has been detrimental to at least one aspect of the industry (eg, turtle farming), it has the benefit of making potential pet owners aware of the risks. This has likely minimized the actual number of zoonotic cases associated with reptiles over the past 2 decades with the resurgence of the pet reptile trade. Zoonotic disease cases could likely be reduced further with common domestic pets if similar broad coverage was given to those animals. Fortunately, it is possible to minimize the potential for zoonotic disease exposure to reptiles and amphibians by following good hygiene and sanitation practices and providing animals an appropriate environment and diet. Although we continue to improve on the latter, it is vastly improved from the days where the incidence of disease (salmonellosis) was considered to be epidemic.

REFERENCES

1. Mitchell MA, Bauer R, Nehlig R, et al. Evaluating the efficacy of Baquacil against *Salmonella* in the aquatic habitat of the red-eared slider (*Trachemys scripta elegans*). J Herp Med Surg 2005;15:9–14.
2. Mitchell MA, Roundtree M. Evaluating the efficacy of polyhexamethylene biguanide at suppressing *Salmonella* Typhimurium in the water column of red-eared sliders (*Trachemys scripta elegans*) under transport. J Herp Med Surg 2006;16:45–8.

3. Mitchell MA, Adamson T, Singleton B, et al. Evaluation of a combination of sodium hypochlorite and polyhexamethylene biguanide as an egg wash for red-eared slider turtles (*Trachemys scripta elegans*) to suppress or eliminate *Salmonella* organisms on egg surfaces and in hatchlings. Am J Vet Res 2007;68:158–64.
4. Zachariah T, Mitchell MA, Serra V, et al. Evaluating the effect of Baquacil® and Sanosil® on *Salmonella* in the aquatic habitat of the red-eared slider turtle (*Trachemys scripta elegans*). J Herp Med Surg 2007;17:76–83.
5. Acha PN, Szyfres B. Salmonellosis. In: Acha PN, Szyfres B, editors. Zoonosis and communicable diseases common to man and animals. 2nd edition. Washington (DC): Pan American Health Organization; 1987. p. 147–55.
6. Smith BP. Salmonellosis. In: Smith BP, editor. Large animal internal medicine. St. Louis: CV Mosby Co; 1991. p. 818–22.
7. Mitchell MA. *Salmonella:* diagnostic methods for reptiles. In: Mader D, editor. Reptile medicine and surgery. St. Louis: Elsevier; 2006. p. 900–5.
8. Lefebvre SL, Reid-Smith R, Boerlin P, et al. Evaluation of the risks of shedding Salmonellae and other potential pathogens by therapy dogs fed raw diets in Ontario and Alberta. Zoonoses Public Health 2008;55:470–80.
9. Lenz J, Joffe D, Kauffman M, et al. Perceptions, practices, and consequences associated with foodborne pathogens and the feeding of raw meat to dogs. Can Vet J 2009;50:637–43.
10. Cherry B, Burns A, Johnson GS, et al. *Salmonella* Typhimurium outbreak associated with veterinary clinic. Emerg Infect Dis 2004;10:2249–51.
11. Van Immerseel F, Pasmans F, De Buck J, et al. Cats as a risk for transmission of antimicrobial drug-resistant *Salmonella*. Emerg Infect Dis 2004;10:2169–74.
12. Swanson SJ, Snider C, Braden CR, et al. Multidrug-resistant *Salmonella enterica* serotype Typhimurium associated with pet rodents. N Engl J Med 2007;356: 21–8.
13. Popoff MY, LeMinor L. Antigenic formulas of the *Salmonella* serovars, 7th revision. Paris (France): World Health Organization Collaborating Center for Reference Research on Salmonella, Pasteur Institute; 1997.
14. McNeil E, Hinshaw WR. *Salmonella* from Galapagos turtles, a Gila monster, and an iguana. Am J Vet Res 1946;7:62–3.
15. Caldwell ME, Ryerson DL. Salmonellosis in certain reptiles. J Infect Dis 1939;65: 242–5.
16. Hinshaw WR, McNeil E. Gopher snakes as carriers of salmonellosis and paracolon infections. Cornell Vet 1944;34:248–54.
17. Boycott JA, Taylor J, Douglas HS. *Salmonella* in tortoises. J Pathol Bacteriol 1953; 65:401–11.
18. Williams LP, Heldson HL. Pet turtles as a cause of human salmonellosis. JAMA 1965;192:347–51.
19. Hersey E, Mason DV. *Salmonella* surveillance report No. 10. Atlanta: US Centers for Disease Control and Prevention; 1963.
20. Lamm SH, Taylor A, Gangarosa EJ, et al. Turtle-associated salmonellosis. I: An estimation of the magnitude of the problem in the United States, 1969–1970. Am J Epidemiol 1972;95:511–7.
21. Altman R, Gorman JC, Bernhardt LL, et al. Turtle-associated salmonellosis. II: The relationship of pet turtles to salmonellosis in children in New Jersey. Am J Epidemiol 1972;95:518–20.
22. Cohen ML, Potter M, Pollard R, et al. Turtle-associated salmonellosis in the United States: effect of public health action 1970–1976. JAMA 1980;243:1247–9.

23. Harris J, Neil KP, Barton Behravesh C, et al. Recent multistate outbreaks of human *Salmonella* infections acquired from turtles: a continuing public health challenge. Clin Infect Dis 2010;50:554–9.
24. Siebling RJ, Neal PM, Granberry WD. Evaluation of methods for the isolation of *Salmonella* and *Arizona* organisms from pet turtles treated with antimicrobial agents. Appl Microbiol 1975;29:240–5.
25. Siebling RJ, Caruso D, Neuman S. Eradication of *Salmonella* and *Arizona* species from turtle hatchlings produced from eggs treated on commercial turtle farms. Appl Environ Microbiol 1984;47:658–62.
26. Shane SM, Gilbert R, Harrington KS. *Salmonella* colonization in commercial pet turtles (*Pseudemys scripta elegans*). Epidemiol Infect 1990;105:307–15.
27. D'Aoust JY, Daley E, Crozier M, et al. Pet turtles: a continuing international threat to public health. Am J Epidemiol 1990;132:233–8.
28. US Centers for Disease Control and Prevention. *Salmonella* survey: annual tabulation summary, 1993–1996. Atlanta: US Centers for Disease Control and Prevention; 1996.
29. Cambre RC, McGuill MW. *Salmonella* in reptiles. In: Bonagura JD, editor. Kirk's current veterinary therapy: XIII small animal practice. Philadelphia: W.B. Saunders; 2000. p. 1185–7.
30. Meehan SK. Swelling popularity. J Am Vet Med Assoc 1996;209:531.
31. Mitchell MA, Shane SM. Preliminary findings of *Salmonella* spp. in captive green iguanas (*Iguana iguana*) and their environment. Prev Vet Med 2000;45:297–304.
32. Cieslak P, Angulo FJ, Dueger EL, et al. Leapin' lizards: a jump in the incidence of reptile-associated salmonellosis. Interscience Conference on Antimicrobial Agents and Chemotherapy, 1994.
33. Ackman DM, Drabkin P, Birkhead G, et al. Reptile-associated salmonellosis in New York state. Pediatric Infect Dis J 1995;14:955–9.
34. Chalker RB, Blaser MJ. A review of human salmonellosis. III: magnitude of *Salmonella* infection in the United States. Rev Infect Dis 1988;10:111–24.
35. Miller RE. American Zoological Association guidelines for animal contact with the general public. Wheeling (WV): American Zoological Association, 1997.
36. Friedman CR, Torigian C, Shillam P, et al. An outbreak of salmonellosis among children attending a reptile exhibit at a zoo. J Pediatrics 1997;132:802–7.
37. Cooke FJ, De Pinna E, Maguire C, et al. First report of human infection with *Salmonella enterica* serovar Apapa resulting from exposure to a pet lizard. J Clin Microbiol 2009;47:2672–4.
38. Tabarani CM, Bennett NJ, Kiska DL, et al. Empyema of preexisting subdural hemorrhage caused by a rare *Salmonella* species after exposure to bearded dragons in a foster home. J Pediatr 2010;156:322–3.
39. US Centers for Disease Control and Prevention. Reptile-associated salmonellosis—selected states, 1998–2002. Morb Mort Wkly Rep 2003;52:1206–9.
40. Bradley Bay T, Angulo FJ. *Salmonella* and reptiles. J Herp Med Surg 2009;19:36–37.
41. US Centers for Disease Control and Prevention. Multistate outbreak of human *Salmonella* Typhimurium infections associated with aquatic frogs—United States, 2009. Morb Mort Wkly Rep 2010;58:1433–6.
42. Harker KS, Lane C, Pinna D, et al. An outbreak of *Salmonella* Typhimurium DT191a associated with feeder mice. Epidemiol Infect 2010;14:1–8.
43. Green SL, Lifland BD, Bouley DM, et al. Disease attributed to *Mycobacterium chelonae* in South African clawed frogs (*Xenopus laevis*). Comp Med 2000;50:675–9.

44. Sanchez-Morgado JM, Gallagher A, Johnson LK. *Mycobacterium gordonae* infection in a colony of African clawed frogs (*Xenopus laevis*). Lab Anim 2009;43:300–3.
45. Hill WA, Newman SJ, Craig L, et al. Diagnosis of *Aeromonas hydrophila*, *Mycobacterium* species, and *Batrachochytrium dendrobatidis* in an African clawed frog (*Xenopus laevis*). J Am Assoc Lab Anim Sci 2010;49:215–20.
46. Karmali MA. Infection by Shiga toxin-producing *Escherichia coli:* an overview. Mol Biotech 2004;26:117–22.
47. Caprioli A, Morabito S, Brugere H, et al. Enterohaemorrhagic *Escherichia coli:* emerging issues on virulence and modes of transmission. Vet Res 2005;36:289–311.
48. Gray MJ, Rajeev S, Miller DL, et al. Preliminary evidence that American bullfrogs (*Rana catesbeiana*) are suitable hosts for *Escherichia coli* O157:H7. Appl Environ Microbiol 2007;73:4066–8.
49. Dipineto L, Gargiulo A, Russo TP, et al. Survey of *Escherichia coli* O157 in captive frogs. J Wildl Dis 2010;46:944–6.
50. Murray BE. Vancomycin-resistant enterococcal infections. N Engl J Med 2000;342: 710–21.
51. Rana SW, Kumar A, Walia SK, et al. Isolation of Tn1546-like elements in vancomycin-resistant *Enterococcus faecium* isolated from wood frogs: an emerging risk for zoonotic bacterial infections to humans. J Appl Microbiol 2010;110:35–43.
52. Mitchell CM, Hutton S, Myers GS, et al. *Chlamydia pneumoniae* is genetically diverse in animals and appears to have crossed the host barrier to humans on (at least) two occasions. PLoS Pathog 2010;695:e1000903.
53. Myers GS, Mathews SA, Eppinger M, et al. Evidence that human *Chlamydia pneumoniae* was zoonotically acquired. J Bacteriol 2009;191:7225–33.
54. Jacobson ER, Telford SR. Chlamydial and poxvirus infections of circulating monocytes of a flap-necked chameleon (*Chamaeleo dilepis*). J Wildl Dis 1990;26:572–7.
55. Homer BL, Jacobson ER, Schumacher J, et al. Chlamydiosis in mariculture-reared green sea turtles (*Chelonia mydas*). Vet Pathol 1994;31:1–7.
56. Huchzermeyer FW, Gerdes GH, Foggin CM, et al. Hepatitis in farmed hatchling Nile crocodiles (*Crocodylus niloticus*) due to chlamydial infection. J S Afr Vet Assoc 1994;65:20–2.
57. Huchzermeyer FW, Langelet E, Putterill JF. An outbreak of chlamydiosis in farmed Indopacific crocodiles (*Crocodylus porosus*). J S Afr Vet Assoc 2008;79:99–100.
58. Jacobson E, Origgi F, Heard D, et al. Immunohistochemical staining of chlamydial antigen in emerald tree boas (*Corallus caninus*). J Vet Diag Invest 2002;14:487–94.
59. Jacobson ER, Heard D, Andersen A. Identification of *Chlamydophila pneumoniae* in an emerald tree boa, *Corallus caninus*. J Vet Diagn Invest 2004;16:153–4.
60. Newcomer CE, Anver MR, Simmons JL, et al. Spontaneous and experimental infections of *Xenopus laevis* with *Chlamydia psittaci*. Lab Anim Sci 1982;32: 680–6.
61. Reed KD, Ruth GR, Meyer JA, et al. *Chlamydia pneumoniae* infection in a breeding colony of African clawed frogs (*Xenopus tropicalis*). Emerg Infect Dis 2000;6: 196–9.
62. Ayinmode A, Adedokun A, Aina A, et al. The zoonotic implications of pentastomiasis in the royal python (*Python regius*). Ghana Med J 2010;44:115–8.
63. Graczyk TK, Cranfield MR, Fayer R. Oocysts of *Cryptosporidium* from snakes are not infectious to ducklings but retain viability after intestinal passage through a refractory host. Vet Parasitol 1998;77:33–40.
64. Griffin C, Reavill DR, Stacy BA, et al. Cryptosporidiosis caused by two distinct species in Russian tortoises and a pancake tortoise. Vet Parasitol 2010;170:14–9.

65. Traversa D, Iorio R, Otranto D, et al. Cryptosporidium from tortoises: genetic characterisation, phylogeny and zoonotic implications. Mol Cell Probes 2008;22:122–8.

66. Schultz H. Human infestation of *Ophionyssus natricis* snake mite. Br J Dermatol 1975;93:695.

67. Nevarez JG, Mitchell MA, Morgan T, et al. Association of West Nile virus with lymphohistiocytic proliferative cutaneous lesions in American alligators (*Alligator mississippiensis*) detected by RT-PCR. J Zoo Wild Med 2008;39:562–6.

Zoonotic Diseases of Common Pet Birds: Psittacine, Passerine, and Columbiform Species

Erika E. Evans, DVM, MBA

KEYWORDS
• Pet • Bird • Zoonoses • Psittacine • Avian • Parrot
• Passerine • Columbiform

Psittacine, passerine, and columbiform birds are among the most popular groups of avian species kept as pets. Fortunately, zoonotic transmission of disease from these species is uncommon, but there are some recognized dangers. Most notably, *Chlamydophila psittaci* can be transmitted from pet birds to humans. *Salmonella* spp, although more commonly a food-borne zoonotic agent, can also be transmitted through pet birds. Allergic responses to pet birds, including pneumonitis and contact dermatitis, have also been documented. Bite wounds from pet birds are rarely reported but can cause trauma and develop infection. The other diseases discussed here are considered potential zoonotic diseases of pet birds because of either isolated reports of suspected but unconfirmed transmission to humans or from reports of wild conspecifics being reported to have the disease. For most diseases, humans with underdeveloped or compromised immune systems, including the very young, the elderly, HIV patients, individuals undergoing chemotherapy, or people otherwise immunosuppressed due to other disease are the most at risk.

BACTERIAL ZOONOSES
Chlamydiosis

Chlamydiosis is a zoonotic disease of great interest to pet bird owners and has received a vast amount of attention. Recently, the National Association of State Public Health Veterinarians (NASPHV) has completed an updated compendium to assist in the prevention and control of chlamydiosis among humans and pet birds.[1] A free copy of the compendium along with other resources to aid pet owners with infected birds, pet stores, and aviaries working toward detection and prevention is available at the NASPHV Web site.[1]

Avian and Zoological Medicine Service, Department of Small Animal Clinical Sciences, College of Veterinary Medicine, University of Tennessee, 2407 River Drive, Knoxville, TN 37996, USA
E-mail address: rikievans@utk.edu

Vet Clin Exot Anim 14 (2011) 457–476
doi:10.1016/j.cvex.2011.05.001
1094-9194/11/$ – see front matter © 2011 Elsevier Inc. All rights reserved.

According to the Centers for Disease Control and Prevention, 66 human cases of psittacosis were reported through the Nationally Notifiable Diseases Surveillance System between 2005 and 2009[1]; these statistics are likely an underrepresentation due to incorrectly diagnosed or unreported cases.[2] Most of the cases reported between 2005 and 2009 were attributed to exposure to pet birds infected with the bacterium.[1] Cockatiels, parakeets, parrots, and macaws were the most commonly represented species. Populations considered to be most at risk include bird owners, pet shop employees, and veterinarians. Due to the zoonotic potential, C psittaci is reportable in most states.

Chlamydiosis is caused by a small bacterial organism called C psittaci.[2–4] This organism is a gram-negative, obligate intracellular bacterium that transitions through at least 2 states during its life cycle. There is an elementary body stage that can infect cells either within the same host or in another host, and a reticulate body stage, which undergoes replication but is not able to infect other cells. An elementary body is extracellular, highly infectious, and metabolically inactive. Elementary bodies are resistant to many environmental stressors and can survive in soil for up to 3 months and in bird droppings for up to 1 month. Elementary bodies are inhaled or ingested by a host and attach themselves to an eukaryotic cell, most commonly a respiratory epithelial cell. After attaching to the cell, the elementary body undergoes endocytosis and forms an endocytoplasmic vesicle. This vesicle allows for the elementary body to remain safe from the host's immune defense system while it undergoes transition into the reticulate body. The reticulate body is the intracellular, metabolically active state that is capable of replication via binary fission. After replication, the reticulate bodies convert to elementary bodies and are released from the cell. Depending on the strain, host, and environmental conditions, the developmental cycle takes 48 to 72 hours. There is also the possibility of a third persistent state in which the organism is present and viable but cannot be eliminated by the host's defense system.[5–6] If this state exists, it is unlikely that a culture could successfully be obtained. The existence of this persistent state is controversial and documentation of its existence in naturally infected birds is lacking.

Birds infected with C psittaci may be asymptomatic.[7,8(pp4–96)] This is especially likely for pigeons and passerine birds, but is also seen with psittacine birds. Stress due to reproduction, raising young, transportation, shipping, overcrowding, and inadequate husbandry can increase the likelihood that birds will begin shedding the organism and/or showing clinical signs. Immunosuppressed birds and very young birds are most likely to succumb to severe infection. The organism can be transmitted vertically, and the very young may die soon after hatching or while still in the nest.

The typical incubation period is anywhere from 3 days to several weeks, but clinical signs and active disease may appear without any known risk or exposure.[1] Many of the clinical signs seen in birds, such as lethargy, decreased appetite, weight loss, and ruffled feathers, are very nonspecific. Disease of the respiratory, gastrointestinal, and ocular systems may result in more visible clinical signs. Liver disease due to C psittaci commonly results in lime-green diarrhea or bright green urates. Conjunctivitis, dyspnea, and ocular and nasal discharge are often reported. Severely affected birds may become completely anorexic, depressed, and die. These clinical signs are not unique to chlamydiosis but may support a potential diagnosis.

When a person becomes infected with C psittaci due to contact with a psittacine bird, the disease process is called psittacosis and has historically been referred to as parrot fever.[9] If a person becomes infected with C psittaci as a result of contact with a nonpsittacine bird, the term ornithosis is applied. Chlamydiosis is a broader term that includes both psittacosis and ornithosis. All of these terms are used somewhat interchangeably in publications regarding zoonoses.

Psittacosis occurs in multiple age groups, but the most severe manifestations of infection are reported in people aged between 35 and 55 years.[4] Children rarely show severe signs when infected, and many individuals shown to be infected with the bacterium show signs mild enough to require minimal to no treatment. The severity of symptoms in people affected with C psittaci can range from subclinical to sepsis with multiorgan failure. Many resources describe flulike symptoms such as fever, chills, headache, muscle aches, and a dry cough as symptoms of human infection with C psittaci. Headache is the most commonly reported sign, followed by cough, dyspnea, confusion, and abnormal liver tests. Pneumonia diagnosed via thoracic radiographs is also commonly reported. The vast majority of people infected with C psittaci show mild signs, and when medical assistance is needed can be treated readily with antibiotic therapy.

There are other less common, more severe expressions of the disease, such as renal complications, hepatitis, pancreatitis, and reactive arthritis.[4] Neurologic and cardiac manifestations are also reported. Some infected individuals develop meningoencephalitis, with the most frequent clinical findings being fever, headache, and confusion. Less commonly, status epilepticus, localized cerebellar ataxia, and brainstem encephalitis are also seen. Cardiac manifestations of the disease include endocarditis, myocarditis, and pericarditis. Symptoms are often present for several months prior to a diagnosis. Endocarditis can be complicated by the development of glomerulonephritis, and surgery is often required even with appropriate and timely antibiotic therapy. Surgical intervention for infective endocarditis is aimed at removing infected tissue, draining any abscesses, repairing heart tissue damaged from the infection, and repairing or replacing affected valves.[10] Mortality with this syndrome approaches 50%.[4] Few other specific clinical presentations have been described in humans, which fortunately are very infrequent, including a fulminant form of psittacosis, gestational psittacosis, and chronic follicular meningitis.[4]

Psittaciforms, passeriforms, and columbiforms are among the 30 bird orders in which C psittaci has been documented.[11] Of these 3 orders of birds, most human cases are associated with exposure to psittacine birds, but passerine birds and columbiform birds are also recognized as sources of human infection.[4] Risk of transmission increases with close contact with infected birds that are actively shedding the organism. Birds undergoing stressful situations such as shipping, overcrowding, reproduction, or malnutrition are more likely to shed, resulting in transmission.[1] Birds that are shedding may not show any sign of disease. Infection is acquired through inhalation of aerosolized organisms in dried feces or respiratory tract secretions and through direct contact with infected birds. Persons developing persistent flulike symptoms, headache, respiratory distress, fever, confusion, or cough should consult with a physician and provide details regarding their exposure and interaction with birds.[4]

A combination of tests, including culture, antibody detection, and antigen detection, are recommended when looking for evidence of infection with C psittaci infection in birds.[1] Infection can be difficult to detect, especially in asymptomatic birds. There are no pathognomonic lesions that can be viewed on gross necropsy, but cloudy air sacs and enlargement of the spleen and liver support a diagnosis of psittacosis. Tissues or impression smears undergoing chromatic or immunologic staining can sometimes aid in identifying organisms. Liver and spleen are preferred tissues for bacterial culture.

In birds showing clinical signs, the use of a combined conjunctival, choanal, and cloacal swab sample and/or liver biopsy can be used for bacteriologic culture or

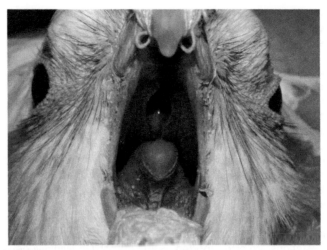

Fig. 1. Sample collection for diagnostic tests, such as bacterial culture and PCR, often includes swabbing the choana of a bird.

polymerase chain reaction (PCR; **Fig. 1**).[1] Depending on the stage of infection and affected tissue, birds may not shed detectable levels of the bacterium in their feces, and for this reason the conjunctival and choanal swabs are preferred to feces. If feces must be used, multiple collections of feces over 3 to 5 consecutive days should be collected and submitted together as a single sample. Samples should be refrigerated after collection and shipped on ice, but not frozen. The individual requirements of each lab may differ, and the sampler is encouraged to contact individual laboratories for their requirements since reliable detection of the bacterium relies heavily on appropriate handling and processing of the samples.

Antibody tests are also available.[1,12] Elementary-body agglutination detects IgM antibody, an early indicator of infection, to the infectious from of *C psittaci* elementary bodies. Indirect fluorescent antibody detects polyclonal secondary antibodies from the host, primarily IgG. Complement fixation is a very sensitive test for antibody but has been associated with a high rate of false-positives in parakeets, young African greys, and lovebirds.[1]

A positive test may reflect either an active infection or an appropriate immunologic response to a previous infection.[12] Antibody might not be found in infected birds that have been acutely infected and are not yet mounting a detectable immune response. Antimicrobial treatment could result in undetectable antibodies, but IgG can persist after successful treatment. To confirm a diagnosis of chlamydiosis, a positive antibody titer must be paired with either 1) a second antibody titer showing at least a fourfold or greater increase in titer, or 2) antigen identification.[1] A positive antibody titer with an elevated white blood cell count, increased serum liver enzymes, and known exposure is not a definitive diagnosis, but are all highly suggestive of chlamydiosis.

Antigen testing detects the presence of the organism even when it is not alive.[1,11] Cross reacting antigens may result in false-positives, and false-negatives can occur when the sample doesn't contain sufficient antigen, which may be due to intermittent shedding. Commercially available antigen tests include enzyme-linked immunosorbent assay and fluorescent antibody test. Positive antigen results should always be evaluated with respect to the presence or absence of clinical signs in the bird. If the bird is asymptomatic, verification that the bird is shedding the organism can be pursued via isolation of the organism.

PCRs are available for testing on combined conjunctival, choanal, and cloacal swab specimens or blood.[1,13] PCR can be very sensitive and specific, but there are no standardized PCR primers and techniques for handling, and processing samples vary. A list of laboratories that currently offer testing for human and avian samples are listed in the NASPHV's compendium on avian chlamydiosis.[1] PCR and culture for avian samples are available at the Diagnostic Center for Population and Health at Michigan State University (Lansing, MI, USA), the Infectious Diseases Laboratory at the University of Georgia College of Veterinary Medicine (Athens, GA, USA), and Texas Veterinary Medical Diagnostic Laboratory (College Station, TX, USA). Some of these laboratories also offer antibody tests for avian samples. The Comparative Pathology Laboratory at the University of Miami (Miami, FL, USA) offers enzyme-linked immunosorbent assay, indirect fluorescent antibody, and PCR, whereas the Diagnostic Virology Lab of the National Veterinary Services Laboratories (Ames, IA, USA), offers culture and complement fixation. NASPHV recommends any birds that are suspected to be infected with C psittaci be evaluated using more than 1 type of test and that all tests are interpreted with regard to the bird's history and clinical signs.

Some veterinarians suggest treating any birds that may be infected regardless of test results, because of the zoonotic risk, but NASPHV discourages prophylactic antibiotic treatment.[1] Currently there is no documentation of antibiotic resistance to C psittaci in birds, but antibiotic resistance has been reported to other Chlamydophila species and is therefore of potential concern.[14] Historically, the treatment of choice was considered to be doxycycline administration for a minimum of 45 days in most species and 30 days in budgerigars.[1] Treatment for this length of time is still recommended to avoid incomplete resolution of infection. However, recent studies have indicated that other less lengthy protocols may be efficacious.[15]

Information regarding dosing and recipes for food and water administration to birds are readily available in the compendium on avian chlamydiosis by NASPHV.[1] Medicated food has successfully been used to treat chlamydiosis in budgerigars and cockatiels.[16,17] Suggested concentrations of doxycycline hyclate medicated water are available for use in cockatiels, African grey parrots, and Goffin's cockatoos.[1] Exotic doves have also been successfully treated using doxycycline-medicated water.[18] Budgerigars do not maintain therapeutic concentrations using medicated water and should be provided the medication via an alternative route. Some birds may develop toxicosis in response to doxycycline. If toxicosis is suspected, treatment with doxycycline should be discontinued and supportive care provided. Treatment can later be attempted with either a reduced dose of doxycycline or alternative regimen.

Pharmacokinetic studies have been undertaken to determine if the use of other medications or decreasing the length of administration of doxycycline from the recommended 45 days may be effective. Oral administration of azithromycin given every 48 hours or doxycycline given every 24 hours for a 21-day course of treatment have both been shown to be effective in treating cockatiels experimentally infected with C psittaci.[15] These results have not yet been tested in naturally infected cockatiels or any other bird species and therefore cannot yet replace the 45-day recommended treatment. Primary motivation to reduce the required length of treatment is to increase the likelihood of owner compliance and therefore decrease recurrence of the disease.

Regardless of which treatment protocol is utilized, infected birds should be isolated from other animals in clean, uncrowded cages.[1] Appropriate husbandry with adequate nutrition and clean water should be maintained to reduce the risk of secondary infection. Birds should be weighed every 3 to 7 days, and if not able to maintain their weight, supplemental and gavage feeding may be required. High dietary intake of calcium from mineral blocks and cuttlebones should be avoided since it can inhibit the absorption of oral tetracyclines. In hand-fed neonates that require supplementation, calcium and tetracyclines should be given at least 4 to 6 hours apart. Facilities should be thoroughly cleaned and disinfected before termination of treatment to reduce the risk of reinfection. Two weeks after the completion of treatment is the earliest suggested time period for repeat screening.

Birds that are sick should not be sold or purchased.[1] Birds from multiple origins should not be combined without proper quarantine (minimum 30 days) and multi-modal testing (antibody, antigen, PCR) for the presence of C psittaci. Cages, food containers, and water bowls should be positioned and cleaned to avoid the spread of fecal matter, feather dander, contaminated food, and other substances between cages. Fecal material and discharged food items should be removed daily. Prior to removal, it is recommended that fecal material and contaminated cage items be wetted or sprayed down to avoid aerosolization of the material. Ventilation should be sufficient to avoid accumulation and limit spread of aerosolized organisms.

In multibird households or facilities, healthy birds should be cared for prior to treatment and/or handling of infected birds.[19] All debris and fecal material should be scrubbed from cages. Disinfectants should be used to thoroughly clean any cages that have housed infected birds before they are reused. Bleach and water at a 1:32 dilution (1/2 cup of 5% chlorine bleach in a gallon of water), 1% Lysol, and quaternary ammonia compounds have been recommended as effective disinfectants. Most disinfectants require at least 5 to 10 minutes of contact time and any items that cannot be properly disinfected should be discarded. Rinse thoroughly to avoid irritation from the detergent. Cleaning methods that limit the aerosolization of materials, such as spraying down cages and floors prior to sweeping and mopping should be used. Vacuum cleaners and pressure washers should be avoided because of the risk of aerosolization.

Once clinical signs are noted in birds and a diagnosis of chlamydiosis obtained, human contact and the potential for transmission has likely already occurred. Therefore, any individuals caring for or surrounded by birds should be made aware of the potential zoonotic risk. People cleaning cages or handling infected birds should wear protective clothing that covers the hands, eyes, and head. These individuals should be fitted with respirators of a N95 or higher rating. When potentially infected birds are necropsied, the procedure should be completed in a biological safety cabinet, and detergent and water should be used to avoid infectious particles becoming aerosolized.

Salmonellosis

Another zoonotic bacterium with reported cases of suspected bird to human transmission is Salmonella.[20] There are 2 species of Salmonella with thousands of different serovars.[21,22] There are some serovars of Salmonella that are specifically adapted for avian hosts, such as Salmonella Pullorum and Salmonella Gallinarum, which primarily cause systemic disease in poultry.[23] Certain strains of Salmonella Typhimurium have been identified as being host adapted for causing disease in pigeons.[24] Salmonella infections with various serovars have been documented in psittacine, passerine, and columbiform birds.[25–27]

Several factors will dictate the manifestation and severity of Salmonella infection in pet birds.[23,28] The ability of the bird to mount an effective immune response will depend on the infecting serovar, age of the animal, and presence of concurrent infection, malnutrition, poor husbandry, or stress, which may increase the risk of severe and potentially fatal infection. Some serovars of *Salmonella*, such as *S* Typhimurium or *Salmonella* Enteritidis are more likely to cause severe illness in both birds and humans.

Salmonella has been shown to have the potential to infect multiple avian organs of the respiratory, gastrointestinal, renal, neurologic, cardiovascular, and reproductive systems.[29(pp953–6)] Clinical signs reported in psittacine birds range from mild enteritis to severe anorexia, diarrhea, lethargy, dehydration, and crop stasis or sudden death. *Salmonella* spp have also been isolated from asymptomatic birds. Suspected transmission of *Salmonella* Typhimurium from psittacine birds to humans has been documented.[9,30–31]

Pigeons infected with *Salmonella* spp may also show a wide variation in clinical signs.[26] Infected pigeons may be asymptomatic and therefore the introduction of new birds, exposure to feral birds, or the routine racing and showing of pigeons carries risk of exposure. In the United Kingdom, where pigeon racing and showing is common, any isolates of *Salmonella* spp obtained from racing and show pigeons must be reported to Animal Health due to zoonotic risk. Pigeons that have ingested the bacterium may show signs of bacteremia and sepsis. Decreased appetite, weight loss, and decreased egg production and viability are commonly seen. Some birds may develop swollen and warm joints from septic or infectious arthritis or exhibit evidence of central nervous system disease.

Wild passerines, both ill and asymptomatic, have been repeatedly documented as carriers of *Salmonella* spp and have been implicated in the transmission of the bacterium to mammals and to humans.[32,33] As seen with infection in other avian species, *Salmonella* Typhimurium in passerines may manifest as systemic and multiorgan disease.[29(pp953–6)] Granulomas have been observed in the liver, spleen, and ceca. Finches and canaries, 2 of the most popular passerines species kept as pets in the United States, have also been shown to exhibit ocular lesions and osteomyelitis.[34]

Salmonellosis in people is usually the result of food borne illness or direct contact with an infected reptile or amphibian, rather than interaction with a pet bird.[35,36] Some individuals that ingest *Salmonella* spp may have no to mild signs of illness.[37] Most individuals that become ill from ingesting *Salmonella* spp have symptoms for 4 to 7 days. Clinical symptoms include abdominal cramps, headache, fever, nausea, vomiting, and copious watery diarrhea. Occasionally the symptoms may be severe enough that hospitalization in indicated. Rarely, serious complication or death may result from infection. In addition to causing gastrointestinal distress, some patients experience other systemic manifestations of infection with the bacterium, including, but not limited to, arthritis, hepatitis, and neuritis. The very young, the elderly, and people with underlying health issues are most likely to suffer severe disease.

The bacterium is typically spread via fecal to oral transmission but can also be spread through direct contact with infected animals or people.[35] The bacteria may be spread mechanically via contaminated clothing, shoes, equipment, and on rodents such as rats and mice.[26] This disease can also be transmitted vertically into the egg or through crop milk. Food and water contaminated with feces from infected animals, both wild and domestic, is also a potential source of infection.

Definitive diagnosis of salmonellosis requires successful culture of the organism. Antemortem, repeat, or pooled fecal samples are cultured. The use of selective enriched culture media is required, and laboratories must be told that salmonellosis is suspected. The shedding of the bacterium is often intermittent and false-negatives are common. Postmortem, multiple samples from a wide range of tissues should be submitted for culture. In flocks with large die off, multiple birds should be submitted for evaluation.

The severity of the disease presentation dictates the intensity of treatment.[26] Supportive care, including fluids and gavage feeding, may be indicated. Antibiotic use is controversial because resistance is common; if warranted, antibiotic choice is best determined by the result of culture and susceptibility testing. Enrofloxacin and amoxicillin are common choices. Maintaining cleanliness within the cages or lofts and providing clean water and food are essential in allowing for recovery. Length of treatment may last from 10 days to 3 weeks to allow for clearance of the bacteria.

Prevention of *Salmonella* spp infection relies heavily on cleanliness.[37] Appropriate husbandry must be maintained, providing for clean surroundings, clean food and water, and avoiding contact with ill and infected animals. Any materials with infected feces should be removed from the enclosure. Sodium hypochlorite (bleach) at a concentration of 0.05% and alkaline peroxide at a concentration of 1% have been shown to be effective against *Salmonella*.[38] The effectiveness of some disinfectants against *Salmonella* adhered to surfaces or contained within a biofilm may be reduced.[39] Suggestions for disinfectants to combat *Salmonella* in these situations include those containing 70% ethanol. Virkon S was also effective at eliminating *Salmonella* found on surfaces. Rodent control should be implemented.[26] Humans working with animals that may carry *Salmonella* spp should wear disposable gloves, frequently wash their hands, discard any items sullied with feces, and avoid eating, drinking, or putting hands near the face and mouth without appropriately washing with soap and warm water.[37]

Mycobacteriosis

Mycobacterium spp are Gram positive, aerobic, acid-fast bacillus that infect birds, mammals, and humans.[40] The most commonly isolated *Mycobacterium* spp from pet birds are *Mycobacterium avium* and *Mycobacterium genevense.* Other species of *Mycobacterium* are infrequently identified in pet birds, including *Mycobacterium tuberculosis,* the agent responsible for tuberculosis in people. *M avium* subsp *Hominis suls* has also been diagnosed in a 6-month-old female, blue-fronted Amazon parrot with inappetence, slight emaciation, heavy biliverdinuria, ascites, and melena.[41] This subspecies rarely causes disease in birds, but has been shown to cause severe disease in humans, especially immunocompromised individuals.

Clinical signs of mycobacteriosis in birds vary widely dependent on the *Mycobacterium* spp, resulting in infection, the species of bird affected, the duration and severity of exposure, and the organ system infected.[41] Weight loss is the most consistent finding reported across multiple species. Respiratory disease can occur, but diarrhea, coelomic distension, and poor feathering are more frequently reported.[42] Weight loss and failure to respond to routine antibiotic therapy are commonly documented in pet birds shown to be suffering from mycobacteriosis.

People afflicted with acquired immune deficiency syndrome are commonly afflicted with what is known as the Mycobacterium complex (*M avium* and *Mycobacterium intracellulare*) and are the individuals most likely to develop systemic mycobacteriosis.[40,43–44] The likelihood of infection increases directly with the severity of immunosuppression. Individuals undergoing organ transplant or those experiencing disease resulting in immunosuppression are also at risk. Fever, weight loss, abdominal pain, fatigue, chronic diarrhea, and anemia are reported in people with systemic mycobacteriosis.

Localized disease also occurs in humans including central nervous system infection, boney or soft tissue lesions, cervical lymphadenitis, or endocarditis.[43]

M tuberculosis causes pulmonary disease known as tuberculosis in humans characterized by a persistent cough, chest pain, and coughing up blood and/or sputum.[45] Other signs include weight loss, fatigue, fever, and generalized malaise. Other parts of the human body may also be impacted by this infection including the kidneys, spine, and brain. Tuberculosis was once the leading cause of death in the United States and is still a common fatal illness in other parts of the world. Many individuals who become infected with *M tuberculosis* develop latent infection because their immune systems are able to fight the disease. Latent infections can transition to active infection within the body, causing illness when a person's immune system is not able to fight the infection. Infection can stay latent weeks to several years, and those with suppressed immune systems, such as those with acquired immunodeficiency system, are at increased risk of becoming ill.

Mycobacterium spp are very stable in the environment and can remain in the soil for years.[40] Infection is typically secondary to ingestion of the bacterium, inhalation of the organism, or from introduction of the organism into open cutaneous lesions. *Mycobacterium* organisms are found worldwide and have been isolated from soil, water, animals, birds, and foods. Environmental sources such as contaminated water, food, and soil are considered the most likely sources of infection for people and animals. Possible transmission of *M tuberculosis* from humans to pet birds, including an African grey and a green-winged macaw, has been reported, and there is concern that a pet bird could harbor this organism and serve as a carrier and source of infection to other birds and humans.[46,47] *M tuberculosis* has also been identified in pet passerines.[48] No confirmed transmission of *Mycobacterium* from a bird to a person has been reported.

Characteristic hemogram findings for birds diagnosed with mycobacteriosis include nonregenerative anemia, and leukocytosis with heterophilia and monocytosis.[40] Depending on the organs most affected, lesions may include pulmonary granulomas, enlarged liver, engorged intestinal loops, or boney lesions. A presumptive diagnosis of mycobacteriosis may be made if acid-fast bacilli are detected in biopsy or necropsy specimens. However, mycobacterial culture or polymerase chain reaction analysis is required for definitive diagnosis. Care must be taken when acid-fast organisms are detected in fecal samples, as nonpathogenic acid-fast organisms, including saprophytes, may be present. Due to the prolonged period of time often necessary to culture *Mycobacterium* spp, diagnosis in birds is often based on histological evidence of mycobacteriosis in diseased tissue (liver, spleen, intestine) and PCR.[49]

Therapy is controversial due to the potential for persistent infection, antibiotic resistance, and the zoonotic potential.[40] If owners want to pursue therapy for a pet bird, it is recommended that the veterinarian have owners sign a release that explains the possibility of transmission of *Mycobacterium* from the bird.[50] Successful treatment has been achieved in pet birds with multimodal antibiotic therapy.[40] Several protocols are available with most, including drugs such as clarithromycin or azithromycin, rifampin or rifabutin, and ethambutol. Treatment takes many months, and monitoring success of treatment is difficult as the organism can be difficult to detect in low numbers.

Reports of transmission of *Mycobacterium* spp to humans from pet birds is lacking. However, there is a recognized potential for human transmission with pet birds potentially serving as reservoirs. Prevention of mycobacteriosis relies heavily on prompt detection of the bacterium and avoiding humans and birds that are showing signs of illness. Maintaining overall health through proper diet and exercise supports a healthy immune system that reduces risk of infection. Making sure that food, water, and the environment are free of contamination can aide in prevention. *Mycobacterium* spp can be challenging to destroy and are often resistant to commonly used disinfectants.[51] Bleach, one of the most commonly used disinfectants is only effective at high concentrations and quaternary ammoniums are not effective. Phenolics are the best disinfectant for inactivating *M tuberculosis* and potentially other *Mycobacterium* spp. Care must be taken to avoid generating droplets or aerosols when cleaning, as inhalation is a primary means of transmission. If a person believes that they or their bird have been exposed to individuals infected with *Mycobacterium* spp they should seek medical or veterinary attention respectively.

Other Bacteria

There are multiple other potential bacterial zoonotic pathogens, including *Mycoplasma,* a bacterium characterized by the lack of a cell wall, which causes conjunctivitis, tracheitis, air sacculitis, and chronic respiratory disease most commonly in poultry and wild passerines, but also in pet birds.[52] Multiple gram-negative bacteria such as *Pasteurella* spp, *Klebsiella* spp, *Yersinia* spp, *Campylobacteriosis* spp, and *Escherichia coli* are also potential zoonotic pathogens identified in pet birds. Documented evidence of zoonotic transmission to humans from pet birds is lacking for these bacterial pathogens but the potential is present. Appropriate hygiene and husbandry, quarantine of sick birds, and maintaining clean food and water sources will reduce risk of infection and possible transmission.

Viral Zoonoses

Avian paramyxovirus, avian influenza, and West Nile virus (WNV) are potential zoonotic infectious agents found in pet bird species. There are not currently any documented cases of direct transmission of these viruses from pet birds to humans, but pet birds have the potential to serve as reservoirs for viral infection. Poultry and wild bird populations, which are discussed elsewhere in this publication, are more likely to harbor these viruses, and therefore, discussion of these viruses within this chapter on pet birds will be abbreviated.

Newcastle Disease Virus

Avian paramyxoviruses (APMV) have been observed in pet birds, but most published descriptions of APMV are based on poultry. APMV includes Newcastle disease virus (NDV), which is caused by serotype 1 (APMV-1).[53] There are nine serovars of avian paramyxovirus, and each serotype is characterized by the type of bird affected. PMV-1 is of great concern in the poultry industry and is a potential zoonotic disease. In humans, NDV infection may result in mild flulike symptoms, conjunctivitis, or laryngitis. Classic Newcastle disease was observed to infect pigeons during poultry outbreaks in the United Kingdom.[26] There is documentation that imported psittacine birds may carry APMV, and passerines have also been shown to suffer from avian paramyxovirus.[54–56] Pigeons may become infected with a variant strain similar—but distinct from—the classic NDV, which is often referred to as PMV-1 or PPMV-1.[26] Monoclonal antibodies are utilized to differentiate this strain from classic exotic Newcastle disease. Vaccination of pigeons for PMV-1 is now a requirement for show and racing pigeons in the United Kingdom.

The virus is shed through respiratory secretions and feces, and exposure to NDV is usually due to ingestion or inhalation of contaminated substances.[53] Direct transmission is possible, and vectors such as insects, humans, and rodents can exacerbate the extent of infection. To confirm a diagnosis, isolation of the virus from infected tissues to identify serotype and virulence must be completed. Antemortem samples typically include cloacal and tracheal swabs. In birds, treatment is supportive and most cases are fatal. Prevention through use of personal protective equipment and good husbandry practices is encouraged to avoid infection.

Influenza

Avian influenza or influenza A is in the family Orthomyxoviridae and has been associated with respiratory disease in multiple avian species, mammals, and humans.[57] There is great variance in clinical signs dependent on the strain and associated virulence and the susceptibility of the infected species.[58] The virus is classified according to surface proteins called hemagglutinin (H) and neuraminidase (N); there are 16 H and 9 N unique proteins currently identified. Many wild birds, especially waterfowl, infected with the virus are asymptomatic and serve as a reservoir for a strain that may result in disease in domestic birds. A highly pathogenic strain, H5N1, has caused significant poultry losses and human disease and death predominantly in Asia over the past decade. This virulent strain also caused death in birds that are typically reservoirs for the virus, including free-ranging ducks, shorebirds, and passerines.[59]

Mild to severe respiratory signs are often accompanied by depression, anorexia, diarrhea, or neurologic signs in birds.[58] Inhalation or direct contact with respiratory, fecal, or ocular secretions are the main modes of transmission.[58,59] Antemortem diagnosis is conducted via viral isolation from tracheal and/or cloacal swabs.[58] Vaccinations are available for birds and have been used in an effort to protect some valuable zoological species of birds; however, due to the potential zoonotic and economic impact, there are strict legal restrictions governing their use.[60] Potential disadvantages of the use of the vaccine include the masking of clinical signs of infection, which could translate into human exposure and possible infection.

There are no current reports of H5N1 in pet birds within the United States; however, there is a report of low pathogenic H5N2 isolated from a 3-month-old red-lored Amazon parrot with severe lethargy and gastrointestinal distress, including regurgitation and melena.[61] The bird was kept in quarantine, given supportive care, and recovered from clinical signs within 4 days. The bird was released 9 weeks after presentation when virus isolation and PCR were negative for the previously identified virus. Avian influenza subtypes H5 and H7 are reportable in the United States, and most often result in depopulation within the poultry industry due to the risk of the virus mutating into a highly pathogenic form. However, as demonstrated in the aforementioned case, not all pet birds are destroyed.

Precautions recommended by the US Department of Agriculture can be taken to protect pet birds from acquiring infectious diseases such as Newcastle disease and avian influenza.[62] First, owners should limit access to their pets. Allowing contact with individuals whom own their own birds, have exposure to sick birds, or work in occupations dealing with birds such as pet stores or poultry plants should be avoided. Owners should make sure their hands and clothes are clean prior to handling their pets. Food and water should be replaced daily. Cages should be kept clean and droppings removed from any toys or materials kept within the household prior to disinfection. If acquiring a new pet bird, proof that the bird was legally imported or bred within the United States should be requested from the seller. Sick birds should never be purchased and new birds should be quarantined for at least 30 days. If a pet bird has been to a show, club meeting, or other event involving exposure to multiple birds, that pet should be kept separate from any other birds in the household for at least 2 weeks. Any birds showing signs of illness should be examined, and multiple deaths within a pet bird collection should be reported to the U.S. Department of Agriculture.

WNV

WNV is a flavivirus for which wild birds have been identified as the main reservoir.[63] The virus causes neurologic and ocular disease in birds and has been associated with neurologic and respiratory manifestations in mammals including humans. The virus was first identified in 1999 in the Western Hemisphere, where wild and zoo birds in the New York City area started dying from the virus. Species commonly kept as pets, including passerine and psittacine birds, have been fatally infected with WNV and may serve as a potential reservoir for human infection.[64,65]

Mosquitoes, primarily *Culex* spp, are the primary route of transmission.[63,64,66] The mosquito becomes infected when feeding on birds infected with the virus and then spreads the virus to mammals, including humans, when the mosquito bites. Oral transmission of the virus through ingestion of infected food items or from direct bird to bird contact as occurs in courtship behavior has been reported. Direct contact, organ transplant, intrauterine contact, and receiving blood donation products have been documented as transmission routes in human infections.

Infected birds often display varying degrees of neurologic compromise, including recumbency and paralysis of the pelvic and thoracic limbs. Virus isolation is best achieved from the brain, spleen, and kidneys. PCR is available and typically performed on oral or cloacal swabs, but is not always successful in antemortem diagnosis.

Clinical symptoms in humans develop 3 to 14 days after being bitten by an infected mosquito. Approximately 80% of people infected with WNV will show no symptoms.[67] Up to 20% of people will show mild signs including fever, headache, nausea, vomiting, and rash. Clinical signs can last for days to weeks. Rarely severe clinical signs such as high fever, neck stiffness, disorientation, tremors, convulsions, weakness, vision loss, numbness, and paralysis may occur. The duration of illness may last weeks and neurologic detriments may be permanent.

Treatment for infection with WNV is primarily supportive. There is no specific treatment, and in birds, infection severe enough to result in neurologic impairment is often fatal. Minor clinical signs identified in people such as fever and muscle aches may pass without any therapy. Severe cases of infection in humans will require hospitalization, intravenous fluid therapy, breathing assistance, and additional supportive care.

Limiting exposure to mosquitoes is the primary goal in prevention. Standing water and areas that promote insect breeding should be treated with larvicides. People should wear repellents when outdoors. Poultry houses and other avian enclosures, including aviaries for zoological species and pet birds, should be constructed to limit insect exposure. Many facilities within the United States that keep captive avian species have started vaccination programs using a commercially available equine vaccine, but efficacy is unknown.[58] Due to concerns over safety and efficacy, vaccination for WNV is not routinely done for pet birds but may be considered in pet birds kept outside with exposure to wild birds and mosquitoes.

Fungal Zoonoses

There are multiple fungal organisms that can infect both birds and humans.[68] *Aspergillus* spp and *Candida* spp are frequently responsible for respiratory or gastrointestinal illness in pet birds, respectively, and can also result in severe disease in immunocompromised individuals. There is currently no evidence that humans acquire these fungal infections directly from birds, but rather acquire infections from environmental exposure.

Some fungal organisms, including *Cryptococcus* spp and *Histoplasmosis* spp, grow well in soil with high nitrogen levels, which is often due to the presence of bird and/or bat feces. *Histoplasmosis capsulatum* is most commonly associated with dove and pigeon feces, and the avoidance of areas that contain high levels of bird and bat droppings are recommended. In most cases, infection with these organisms goes unnoticed and humans are asymptomatic. In a few cases, symptoms of respiratory disease, including cough, headache, chest pain, and fever, can result. In rare cases, histoplasmosis can become disseminated and spread to organs outside the lungs. *Cryptococcus neoformans* has a tendency to infect the central nervous system and can result in meningoencephalitis. When symptoms are severe or the person is immunocompromised, infection without appropriate antifungal treatment can be fatal.

Birds rarely develop clinical signs associated with colonization of *C neoformans*. There is one report of a Moluccan cockatoo suffering from systemic cryptococcal disease and one report of a cockatoo that exhibited cutaneous lesions.[69,70] Human infection with these organisms is not from direct transmission from a bird, but rather from exposure to the organisms in the environment, and therefore—strictly speaking—is not considered zoonotic. However, some of these fungal organisms may be found in the feces of caged birds and therefore, pet birds may serve as a potential reservoir for infection.[71–75] Individuals who are immunocompromised are considered at risk, and rarely, otherwise healthy individuals may become ill from infection with *Cryptococcus* spp.[76]

There are 2 reports of meningitis from *C neoformans* in the literature that are believed to be due to exposure to a pet bird's contaminated and aerosolized excreta. An elderly, immunocompromised woman was diagnosed with meningitis from an isolate of *C neoformans* identical to one recovered from the feces of an asymptomatic Umbrella cockatoo cared for in the same household.[77] Exposure to aerosolized cockatoo excreta containing *C neoformans* was cited as the suspected cause of human infection. Although the bird had shared the same home with the woman for 7 years, the bird was housed on a different floor of the house and the woman was not directly involved in caring for the bird or cleaning its cage. In the second case, an immunocompetent woman was diagnosed with *Cryptococcus* meningitis after exposure to a magpie bird kept as a pet in her parent's household.[78] The magpie's feces cultured positive for *C neoformans.* No direct contact with the bird was identified and the woman had only lived in the house with the bird for 3 months. Consistent with the suspected aerosol exposure described in these cases, experimentally, *C neoformans* has successfully been isolated from air near caged birds.[79] Cutaneous nodular lesions due to dermatologic infection with *Cryptococcosis* spp have also been observed in an immunocompromised pet cockatoo owner, but the origin of the infection was not published.[80]

Parasitic Zoonoses

Species of birds kept as pets have been diagnosed with *Giardia* spp and *Cryptosporidium* spp.[81–83] However, to the author's knowledge there are no reports of direct transmission from a pet bird to a human in the literature. There are reports of wild birds serving as possible reservoirs for the parasites, increasing the possibility of pet birds also serving as reservoirs.[84–89]

Most *Giardia* spp isolated from birds, such as *Giardia ardeae* and *Giardia psittaci* are not considered zoonotic due to their host specificity.[81] However, 1 species isolated from psittacine birds, *Giardia duodenalis* may be infectious to humans. *G duodenalis* trophozoites isolated from a parrot (*Cacatua galerita*) were used to colonize the small intestinal tracts of domestic kittens and lambs.[90] The experimental infection resulted in diarrhea in most of the kittens, but the lambs remained asymptomatic. This indicates that this *Giardia* sp may infect some pet bird species, resulting in a potential source of infection and disease for some mammals, potentially including humans.

Cryptosporidium spp reside in the gastrointestinal system of infected humans and animals.[91] The organism can be passed in droppings, and contaminated water is the most frequently cited source of infection. Research indicates that wild birds including songbirds, parrots, and pigeons may be a mechanical vector for this parasite, increasing the risk of pet bird and human exposure.[75,81–83]

Ectoparasites found on birds have the potential to cause dermatologic lesions in humans.[20] Mites, including *Ornithonyssus sylviarum* and *Dermanyssus gallinae,* most commonly infect poultry and wild birds and are very rare in pet birds.[92] Human skin serves as an incidental host and lesions are mostly localized, but can be intensely pruritic. Papular to papulovesicular eruptions in response to the mite can also occur. These mites cannot reproduce on a human host and thus, the infection is self-limiting. The sections of this publication focusing on zoonotic infections from poultry and wild bird populations should be consulted for additional information.

Hypersensitivities and Dermatologic Conditions

Hypersensitivity pneumonitis (HP) is a lung disease characterized by lymphocytic inflammation and formation of granulomatous pulmonary lesions resulting from an inhaled antigen.[93] Dust and mites encountered during occupational exposure have historically been the most frequently cited antigens, however case reports of HP resulting from exposure to pet birds, including psittacine and columbiform species, are increasing in frequency. Exposure to feathers, feather dander, and bird droppings have all been linked to allergic alveolitis. In addition to pet bird exposure, bedding filled with feathers from species of waterfowl and poultry has also been implicated in causing HP.

There are documented reports of pet birds suffering from a suspected similar allergic pneumonitis.[94] Most instances involve South American psittacine birds exposed to the feather dander in the environment from another avian species, most notably cockatoos and cockatiels. This disease is commonly called chronic obstructive pulmonary disease or macaw pulmonary hypersensitivity because of the over-representation of blue and gold macaws (*Ara ararauna*).[95] Although early stages of the disorder often go unnoticed, advanced stages are often characterized by polycythemia and exercise intolerance.[96] Atrial smooth muscle hypertrophy is the most prominent lesion, but proliferation of parabronchial lymphoid tissue and lymphoid nodular formation may also occur. Treatment is based on symptomatic therapy, air purification, and removal of the inciting antigen.

In people, HP can present as either an acute or chronic form.[93,97] The acute form often results in symptoms 4 to 6 hours after exposure to the antigen. Cough, fever, chest pain, dyspnea, and generalized malaise are common symptoms of acute exposure to an antigen to which the individual has hypersensitivity. In the chronic form, signs are more gradual, but often progressive and can include breathlessness that is exacerbated during exercise, a dry cough, decreased appetite, and unplanned weight loss. There may be a genetic predisposition in people that results in the development of HP.[93] Diagnosis is often based on history of antigen exposure, clinical symptoms, blood work, and imaging (including chest radiographs and CT). In some cases bronchoscopy with biopsies, pulmonary function tests, and antibody panels to detect specific hypersensitivities may also be performed. Treatment involves identifying and avoiding the antigen, which can be difficult when the bird is living in the home as a pet. Removal of carpeting, regular cleaning, and air filtration can reduce antigen burdens in the home. For individuals breeding birds, a change in occupation may be necessary. Glucocorticoids may be given to reduce inflammation in the chronic form of the disease. When exposure to the antigen continues and treatment is not initiated, irreversible pulmonary fibrosis and/or emphysema may result.

Birds most commonly reported to be associated with the development of HP include pigeons and budgerigars.[98] It is possible that this overrepresentation may be due to the popularity of these species as pets. Other avian species frequently cared for as pets, including canaries and various other psittacine birds such as cockatiels, lovebirds, and rosella parrots have also been associated with HP in humans.[99,100]

Cutaneous reactions from skin allergies can also result from dermatologic exposure to pet birds.[101] Additionally, as most pet bird owners know, pet birds can bite and cause significant skin lesions. Despite the fact that animal bites are the most commonly documented zoonotic risk from pets, bites and scratches from pet birds are rarely reported in peer-reviewed literature. However, secondary infection developed following a bite from a pet cockatoo in a 68-year-old woman.[102] She was bitten on her right hand between the second and third digits; the woman did not seek professional medical advice until 30 days after the bite occurred. Culture of the lesion was positive for *Mycobacterium chelonae/abscessus*. The wound was surgically excised and long-term antibiotic therapy for 12 months was eventually successful. A second report documents a 59-year-old diabetic woman who was diagnosed with pyoderma gangrenosum after being bitten and scratched by a crow.[103] Pyoderma gangrenosum, a rare noninfectious neutrophilic dermatosis is typically associated with an underlying systemic disease. The initial bite wound cultured positive for *Citrobacter koseri* and *E coli,* both of which have been cultured from the gastrointestinal tract of birds. Although bird bite reports are rare in the literature, the potential for severe tissue damage, infection, and systemic illness exist, and those suffering bites from pet birds should perform appropriate wound care, including cleaning and flushing, and seek medical attention when appropriate. Research is needed to more fully assess the risk associated with bites sustained from pet birds, particularly infection that can occur due to inoculation of bacteria into the wound.

SUMMARY

In summary, true zoonotic infection resulting from exposure to pet birds is rare. Most birds with potentially zoonotic diseases do not present serious risk to healthy individuals, but all individuals interacting with birds should observe proper hygiene practices to lessen the risk of transmission. Individuals handling pet birds or their excretions should ensure proper sanitation. Veterinarians play multiple critical roles in limiting exposure to zoonotic and potentially zoonotic diseases. Routine and preventative veterinary care can aid in the recognition and treatment of disease. By developing a thorough understanding of the diseases and methods of transmission, veterinarians can effectively communicate risks and appropriate precautions to their staff and pet bird owners.

REFERENCES

1. Smith KA, Campbell CT, Murphy J, et al. Compendium of measures to control Chlamydophila psittaci infection among humans (psittacosis) and pet birds (avian chlamydiosis). Available at: http://www.nasphv.org/Documents/Psittacosis.pdf. Accessed February 10, 2011.

2. Centers for Disease Control and Prevention. Psittacosis. Available at: http://www.cdc.gov/ncidod/dbmd/diseaseinfo/psittacosis_t.htm. Accessed February 10, 2011.
3. Vanrompay D, Ducatelle R, Haesebrouck F. Chlamydia psittaci infections: a review with emphasis on avian chlamydiosis. Vet Microbiol 1995;45(2–3):93–119.
4. Stewardson AJ, Grayson ML. Psittacosis. Infect Dis Clin North Am 2010;24(1):7–25.
5. Hogan RJ, Mathews SA, Mukhopadhyay S, et al. Chlamydial persistence: beyond the biphasic paradigm. Infect Immun 2004;72(4):1843–55.
6. Beatty WL, Morrison RP, Byrne GI. Persistent chlamydiae: from cell culture to a paradigm for chlamydial pathogenesis. Microbiol Rev 1994;58(4):686–99.
7. Flammer K. Chlamydia. In: Altman RB, Clubb SL, Dorrestein GM, et al, editors. Avian medicine and surgery. Philadelphia: WB Saunders Co; 1997:364–79.
8. Gerlach H. Chlamydia. In: Ritchie BW, Harrison GJ, Harrison LR, editors. Avian medicine: principles and application. Lake Worth (FL): Wingers Publishing, Inc; 1994.
9. Grimes JE. Zoonoses acquired from pet birds. Vet Clin North Am Small Anim Pract 1987;17(1):209–18.
10. Olaison L, Pettersson G. Current best practices and guidelines. Indications for surgical intervention in infective endocarditis. Cardiol Clin 2003;21(2):235–51.
11. Kaleta EF, Taday EMA. Avian host range of Chlamydophila spp. based on isolation, antigen detection and serology. Avian Pathol 2003;32(5):435–62.
12. Grimes JE, Arizmendi F, Carter CN, et al. Diagnostic serologic testing of cage and aviary birds for chlamydiosis and suggested confirmatory testing. J Vet Diagn Invest 1996;8(1):38–44.
13. Geens T, Dewitte A, Boon N, et al. Development of a Chlamydophila psittaci species-specific and genotype-specific real-time PCR. Vet Res 2005;36(5–6):787–97.
14. Dugan J, Rockey DD, Jones L, et al. Tetracycline resistance in Chlamydia suis mediated by genomic islands inserted into the chlamydial inv-like gene. Antimicrob Agents Chemother 2004;48(10):3989–95.
15. Guzman DS, Diaz-Figueroa O, Tully T Jr, et al. Evaluating 21-day doxycycline and azithromycin treatments for experimental Chlamydophila psittaci infection in cockatiels (Nymphicus hollandicus). J Avian Med Surg 2010;24(1):35–45.
16. Flammer K, Trogdon MM, Papich M. Assessment of plasma concentrations of doxycycline in budgerigars fed medicated seed or water. J Am Vet Med Assoc 2003;223(7):993–8.
17. Powers LV, Flammer K, Papich M. Preliminary investigation of doxycycline plasma concentrations in cockatiels (Nymphicus hollandicus) after administration by injection or in water or feed. J Avian Med Surg 2000;14(1):23–30.
18. Padilla LR, Flammer K, Miller RE. Doxycycline-medicated drinking water for treatment of Chlamydophila psittaci in exotic doves. J Avian Med Surg 2005;19(2):88–91.
19. National Association of State Public Health Veterinarians. Psittacosis and avian chlamydiosis checklist for owners of infected birds. Available at: http://www.nasphv.org/Documents/PsittacosisChecklistOwners.pdf. Accessed February 10, 2011.
20. Jorn KS, Thompson KM, Larson JM, et al. Polly can make you sick: pet bird-associated diseases. Cleve Clin J Med 2009;76(4):235–43.
21. Brenner FW, Villar RG, Angulo FJ, et al. Salmonella nomenclature. J Clin Microbiol 2000;38(7):2465–7.
22. Heyndrickx M, Pasmans F, Ducatelle R, et al. Recent changes in Salmonella nomenclature: the need for clarification. Vet J 2005;170(3):275–7.

23. Lister SA, Barrow P. Enterobacteriaceae. In: Pattison M, McMullin PF, Bradbury JM, et al, editors. Poultry diseases. 6th edition. Edinburgh (Scotland): Saunders Elsevier; 2008. p. 110–45.

24. Pasmans F, Van Immerseel F, Heyndrickx M, et al. Host adaptation of pigeon isolates of Salmonella enterica subsp. enterica serovar Typhimurium variant Copenhagen phage type 99 is associated with enhanced macrophage cytotoxicity. Infect Immun 2003;71(10):6068–74.

25. Vigo GB, Origlia J, Gornatti D, et al. Isolation of Salmonella typhimurium from dead blue and gold macaws (Ara ararauna). Avian Dis 2009;53(1):135–8.

26. Pennycott T. Pigeons: infectious diseases. In: Chitty J, Lierz M, editors. BSAVA manual of raptors, pigeons and passerine birds. Quedgeley, Gloucester (England): British Small Animal Veterinary Association; 2008. p. 311–9.

27. Madadgar O, Salehi TZ, Ghafari MM, et al. Study of an unusual paratyphoid epornitic in canaries (Serinus canaria). Avian Pathol 2009;38(6):437–41.

28. Piccirillo A, Mazzariol S, Caliari D, et al. Salmonella Typhimurium phage type DT160 infection in two Moluccan cockatoos (Cacatua moluccensis): clinical presentation and pathology. Avian Dis 2010;54(1):131–5.

29. Gerlach H. Bacteria. In: Ritchie BW, Harrison GJ, Harrison LR, editors. Avian medicine: principles and application. Lake Worth (FL): Wingers Publ., Inc.; 1994. p. 953–6.

30. Harris JM. Zoonotic diseases of birds. Vet Clin North Am Small Anim Pract 1991; 21(6):1289–98.

31. Madewell BR, McChesney AE. Salmonellosis in a human infant, a cat, and two parakeets in the same household. J Am Vet Med Assoc 1975;167(12):1089–90.

32. Morishita TY, Aye PP, Ley EC, et al. Survey of pathogens and blood parasites in free-living passerines. Avian Dis 1999;43(3):549–52.

33. Handeland K, Nesse LL, Lillehaug A, et al. Natural and experimental Salmonella Typhimurium infections in foxes (Vulpes vulpes). Vet Microbiol 2008;132(1–2): 129–34.

34. Joesph V. Infectious and parasitic diseases of captive passerines. Semin Avian Exotic Pet Med 2003;12(1):21–8.

35. Coburn B, Grassl GA, Finlay BB. Salmonella, the host and disease: a brief review. Immunol Cell Biol 2007;85(2):112–8.

36. Owens MD. Salmonella infection in emergency medicine. Available at: http://emedicine.medscape.com/article/785774-print. Accessed February 10, 2011.

37. Centers for Disease Control and Prevention. Salmonella. Available at: http://www.cdc.gov/salmonella/. Accessed February 10, 2011.

38. Ramesh N, Joseph SW, Carr LE, et al. Evaluation of chemical disinfectants for the elimination of Salmonella biofilms from poultry transport containers. Poult Sci Jun 2002;81(6):904–10.

39. Moretro T, Vestby LK, Nesse LL, et al. Evaluation of efficacy of disinfectants against Salmonella from the feed industry. J Appl Microbiol 2009;106(3):1005–12.

40. Lennox AM. Mycobacteriosis in companion psittacine birds: a review. J Avian Med Surg 2007;21(3):181–7.

41. Shitaye EJ, Grymova V, Grym M, et al. Mycobacterium avium subsp. hominissuis infection in a pet parrot. Emerg Infect Dis 2009;15(4):617–9.

42. Campbell T. Mycobacterial tracheitis in a double-yellow-headed Amazon parrot (Amazona ochrocephala oratrix). Exotic Pet Pract 1997;2(1):7.

43. AIDS Education & Training Centers National Resource Center Web site. Available at: http://www.aidsetc.org/. Accessed February 10, 2011.

44. Centers for Disease Control and Prevention. You can prevent MAC (Disseminated mycobacterium avium complex disease). Available at: http://www.cdc.gov/hiv/resources/brochures/mac.htm. Accessed February 10, 2011.

45. Centers for Disease Control and Prevention. Tuberculosis (TB). Available at: http://www.cdc.gov/tb/topic/basics/default.htm. Accessed February 10, 2011.

46. Steinmetz HW, Rutz C, Hoop RK, et al. Possible human-avian transmission of Mycobacterium tuberculosis in a green-winged macaw (Ara chloroptera). Avian Dis 2006;50(4):641–5.

47. Schmidt V, Schneider S, Schlomer J, et al. Transmission of tuberculosis between men and pet birds: a case report. Avian Pathol 2008;37(6):589–92.

48. Hoop RK. Mycobacterium tuberculosis infection in a canary (Serinus canana) and a blue-fronted Amazon parrot (Amazona amazona aestiva). Avian Dis 2002;46(2):502–4.

49. Tell LA, Foley J, Needham ML, et al. Diagnosis of avian mycobacteriosis: comparison of culture, acid-fast stains, and polymerase chain reaction for the identification of Mycobacterium avium in experimentally inoculated Japanese quail (Coturnix coturnix japonica). Avian Dis 2003;47(2):444 62.

50. Babcock S, Marsh AE, Lin J, et al. Legal implications of zoonoses for clinical veterinarians. J Am Vet Med Assoc 2008;233(10):1556–62.

51. Best M, Sattar SA, Springthorpe VS, et al. Efficacies of selected disinfectants against Mycobacterium tuberculosis. J Clin Microbiol 1990;28(10):2234–39.

52. Bradbury JM, Morrow C. Avian mycoplasmas. In: Pattison M, McMullin PF, Bradbury JM, editors. Poultry diseases. 6th edition. Edinburgh (Scotland): Saunders Elsevier; 2008. p. 220–34.

53. Alexander DJ, Jones RC. Paramyxoviridae. In: Pattison M, McMullin PF, Bradbury JM, editors. Poultry diseases. 6th edition. Edinburgh (Scotland): Saunders Elsevier; 2008. p. 294–316.

54. Utterback WW, Schwartz JH. Epizootiology of velogenic viscerotropic Newcastle disease in southern California, 1971–1973. J Am Vet Med Assoc 1973;163(9):1080–8.

55. Pearson GL, McCann MK. The role of indigenous wild, semidomestic, and exotic birds in the epizootiology of velogenic viscerotropic Newcastle disease in southern California, 1972–1973. J Am Vet Med Assoc 1975;167(7):610–4.

56. Senthuran S, Vijayarani K, Kumanan K, et al. Pathotyping of Newcastle disease virus isolates from pet birds. Acta Virologica 2005;49(3):177–82.

57. Mase M, Imada T, Sanada Y, et al. Imported parakeets harbor H9N2 influenza A viruses that are genetically closely related to those transmitted to humans in Hong Kong. J Virol 2001;75(7):3490–4.

58. Stanford M. Raptors: infectious diseases. In: Chitty J, Lierz M, editors. BSAVA manual of raptors, pigeons and passerine birds. Quedgeley, Gloucester (England): British Small Animal Veterinary Association; 2008. p. 212–22.

59. Jones MP. Selected infectious diseases of birds of prey. J Exot Pet Med 2006;15(1):5–17.

60. Philippa J, Baas C, Beyer W, et al. Vaccination against highly pathogenic avian influenza H5N1 virus in zoos using an adjuvanted inactivated H5N2 vaccine. Vaccine 2007;25(19):3800–8.

61. Hawkins MG, Crossley BM, Osofsky A, et al. Avian influenza A virus subtype H5N2 in a red-lored Amazon parrot. J Am Vet Med Assoc 2006;228(2):236–41.

62. U.S. Department of Agriculture, Animal and Plant Health Inspection Services. Protect your pet from bird flu. Available at: http://www.aphis.usda.gov/publications/animal_health/content/printable_version/ProtectYourPetBird2006.pdf. Accessed February 10, 2011.

63. West Nile virus infection in poultry. In: Kahn CM, Line S, Aiello SE, editors. The Merck veterinary manual. 8th edition. Whitehouse Station (NJ): Merck & Co, Inc; 2008.
64. Pollock CG. West Nile virus in the Americas. J Avian Med Surg 2008;22(2):151–7.
65. Carboni DA, Nevarez JG, Tully TN, et al. West Nile Virus infection in a sun conure (Aratinga solstitialis). J Avian Med Surg 2008;22(3):240–5.
66. Sejvar JJ, Bode AV, Marfin AA, et al. West Nile virus-associated flaccid paralysis outcome. Emerg Infect Dis 2006;12(3):514–6.
67. Centers for Disease Control and Prevention. West Nile Virus: what you need to know. 2006; Available at: http://www.cdc.gov/ncidod/dvbid/westnile/wnv_factsheet.htm. Accessed February 10, 2011.
68. Mani I, Maguire JH. Small Animal zoonoses and immuncompromised pet owners. Top Companion Anim Med 2009;24(4):164–74.
69. Fenwick B, Takeshita K, Wong A. A moluccan cockatoo with disseminated cryptococcosis. J Am Vet Med Assoc 1985;187(11):1218–9.
70. Lester SJ, Kowalewich NJ, Bartlett KH, et al. Clinicopathologic features of an unusual outbreak of cryptococcosis in dogs, cats, ferrets, and a bird: 38 cases (January to July 2003). J Am Vet Med Assoc 2004;225(11):1716–22.
71. Abou-Gabal M, Atia M. Study of the role of pigeons in the dissemination of Cryptococcus neoformans in nature. Sabouraudia 1978;16(1):63–8.
72. Criseo G, Bolignano MS, Deleo F, et al. Evidence of canary droppings as as important reservoir of Cryptococcus Neoformans. Int J Med Microbiol Virol Parasitol Infect Dis 1995;282(3):244–54.
73. Staib F, Schulz-Dieterich J. Cryptococcus neoformans in fecal matter of birds kept in cages. Zentralbl Bakteriol Mikrobiol Hyg B 1984;179(2):179–86.
74. Raso TF, Werther K, Miranda E, et al. Cryptococcosis outbreak in psittacine birds in Brazil. Med Mycol 2004;42(4):355–62.
75. Rosario I, Acosta B, Colom F. Pigeons and other birds as a reservoir for Cryptococcus spp. Revista Iberoamericana De Micologia 2008;25(1):S13–8.
76. Terada T. Cryptococcosis in the central nervous system in a 36-year-old Japanese man: an autopsy study. Tohoku J Exp Med 2010;222(1):33–7.
77. Nosanchuk JD, Shoham S, Fries BC, et al. Evidence of zoonotic transmission Cryptococcus neoformans from a pet cockatoo to an immunocompromised patient. Ann Intern Med 2000;132(3):205–8.
78. Lagrou K, Van Eldere J, Keuleers S, et al. Zoonotic transmission of Cryptococcus neoformans from a magpie to an immunocompetent patient. J Intern Med 2005; 257(4):385–8.
79. Staib F. Sampling and isolation of Cryptococcus neoformans from indoor air with the aid of the Reuter Centrifugal Sampler (RCS) and guizotia abyssinica creatinine agar. A contribution to the mycological-epidemiological control of Cr. neoformans in the fecal matter of caged birds. Zentralbl Bakteriol Mikrobiol Hyg B 1985;180(5–6):567–75.
80. Rosen T, Jablon J. Infectious threats from exotic pets: dermatological implications. Dermatol Clin 2003;21(2):229–36.
81. Tsai SS, Hirai K, Itakura C. Histopathological survey of protozoa, helminths, and ascardis of imported and local psittacine and passerine birds in Japan. Jpn J Vet Res 1992;40(4):161–74.
82. Gondim LSQ, Abe-Sandes K, Uzeda RS, et al. Toxoplasma gondii and Neospora caninum in sparrows (Passer domesticus) in the Northeast of Brazil. Vet Parasitol 2010;168(1–2):121–4.
83. Abreu-Acosta N, Foronda-Rodriguez P, Lopez M, et al. Occurrence of Cryptosporidium hominis in pigeons (Columba livia). Acta Parasitologica 2009;54(1):1–5.

84. Kassa H, Harrington BJ, Bisesi MS. Cryptosporidiosis: a brief literature review and update regarding Cryptosporidium in feces of Canada geese (Branta canadensis). J Environ Health 2004;66(7):34–9.
85. Majewska AC, Graczyk TK, Slodkowicz-Kowalsk A, et al. The role of free-ranging, captive, and domestic birds of Western Poland in environmental contamination with Cryptosporidium parvum oocysts and Giardia lamblia cysts. Parasitol Res 2009; 104(5):1093–9.
86. Plutzer J, Tomor B. The role of aquatic birds in the environmental dissemination of human pathogenic Giardia duodenalis cysts and Cryptosporidium oocysts in Hungary. Parasitol Int 2009;58(3):227–31.
87. Schets FA, van Wijnen JH, Schijven JF, et al. Monitoring of waterborne pathogens in surface waters in Amsterdam, The Netherlands, and the potential health risk associated with exposure to Cryptosporidium and Giardia in these waters. Appl Environ Microbiol 2008;74(7):2069–78.
88. Andrzejewska I, Tryjanowski P, Zduniak P, et al. Toxoplasma gondii antibodies in the white stork (Ciconia ciconia). Berlin Munch Tierarztl Wochenschr 2004;117(7–8): 274–5.
89. Leite AS, Alves LC, Faustino MAG. Serological survey of toxoplasmosis in birds from Cracidae family in a wild bird center facility at Pernambuco State, Northeast of Brazil. Medicina Veterinaria-Recife 2007;1(1):55–7.
90. McDonnell PA, Scott KGE, Teoh DA, et al. Giardia duodenalis trophozoites isolated from a parrot (Cacatua galerita) colonize the small intestinal tracts of domestic kittens and lambs. Vet Parasitol 2003;111(1):31–46.
91. Centers for Disease Control and Prevention. Parasites. Available at: http://www.cdc.gov/parasites/. Accessed February 10, 2011.
92. Orton DI, Warren LJ, Wilkinson JD. Avian mite dermatitis. Clin Exp Dermatol 2000;25(2):129–31.
93. Lacasse Y, Cormier Y. Hypersensitivity pneumonitis. Orphanet J Rare Dis 2006;1:25.
94. Tully TN Jr, Harrison GJ. Pneumonology. In: Ritchie BW, Harrison GJ, Harrison LR, editors. Avian medicine: principles and application. Lake Worth (FL): Wingers Publishing, Inc; 1994. p. 556–81.
95. Phalen DN. Respiratory medicine of cage and aviary birds. Vet Clin North Am Exot Anim Pract 2000;3(2):423–52.
96. Reavill DR. The differential diagnosis. Presented at the Association of Avian Veterinarians Conference. Providence (RI), August, 2007.
97. Hoppin JA, Umbach DM, Kullman GJ, et al. Pesticides and other agricultural factors associated with self-reported farmer's lung among farm residents in the Agricultural Health Study. Occup Environ Med 2007;64(5):334–41.
98. Morell F, Roger A, Reyes L, et al. Bird fancier's lung: a series of 86 patients. Medicine (Baltimore) 2008;87(2):110–30.
99. Caruana M, Cornish KS, Bajada S, et al. Rosella parrot exposure as a cause of bird fancier's lung. Arch Environ Occup H 2005;60(4):187–92.
100. Funke M, Fellrath JM. Hypersensitivity pneumonitis secondary to lovebirds: a new cause of bird fancier's disease. Eur Respir J 2008;32(2):517–21.
101. Gorman J, Cook A, Ferguson C, et al. Pet birds and risks of respiratory disease in Australia: a review. Aust N Z J Public Health 2009;33(2):167–72.
102. Larson JM, Gerlach SY, Blair JE, et al. Mycobacterium chelonae/abscessus infection caused by a bird bite. Infect Dis Clin Pract 2008;16(1):60–1.
103. Tripathi AK, Erdmann MWH. Bird-bite infection and pyoderma gangrenosum: a rare combination? J Plast Reconstr Aesthetic Surg 2008;61(11):1409–11.

Zoonoses, Public Health, and the Backyard Poultry Flock

Vanessa L. Grunkemeyer, DVM, DABVP (Avian)

KEYWORDS

• Zoonoses • Avian • Poultry • *Salmonella* • Influenza

ZOONOSES AND NOTIFIABLE DISEASES

Zoonoses are infectious diseases which are directly or indirectly transmitted from animals to humans. Sixty-one percent of the 1415 infectious agents recognized to be pathogenic to humans are zoonotic, among which are multiple bacterial, viral, fungal, and parasitic avian diseases.[1] Confirmed human cases of many of these zoonotic diseases are nationally notifiable. The Centers for Disease Control and Prevention (CDC) list of Nationally Notifiable Diseases includes human salmonellosis, chlamydophilosis, listeriosis, eastern equine encephalitis (EEE), western equine encephalitis (WEE), West Nile virus (WNV), novel influenza A viruses, and cryptosporidiosis.[2,3] Avian cases of *Salmonella pullorum*, *Salmonella gallinarum*, EEE, WNV, influenza, and Chlamydophila are also reportable.[2,4]

Limited information is available about the prevalence of zoonotic diseases in backyard poultry and the relative risk of their transmission to hobby farmers. Due to the extreme differences in husbandry and medical practices between large commercial poultry flocks and small private flocks, it is unknown how accurately information can be extrapolated between the practices. However, veterinarians who treat backyard poultry should be knowledgeable about potential avian zoonotic infections so that they can accurately identify outbreaks. In maintaining an appropriate standard of care, veterinarians also have legal and ethical obligations to educate owners regarding the potential zoonotic diseases carried by their pets, recommend measures to prevent zoonotic disease transmission, and advise owners to seek medical care from a physician in the case of potential zoonotic disease transmission.[5]

GENERAL ZOONOTIC DISEASE PREVENTION RECOMMENDATIONS

The foundations of zoonotic disease prevention are education of owners regarding appropriate flock husbandry and biosecurity, disease identification and control, and personal protection measures to prevent disease transmission to humans.

The author has nothing to disclose.
Department of Clinical Sciences, North Carolina State University College of Veterinary Medicine, 4700 Hillsborough Street, Raleigh, NC 27606, USA
E-mail address: vlg7@cornell.edu

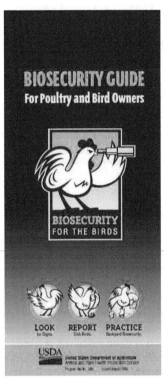

Fig. 1. Biosecurity guide for poultry and bird owners. (*From* United States Department of Agriculture Animal and Plant Health Inspection Service (USDA-APHIS) Biosecurity Guide for Poultry and Bird Owners. Available at: http://www.aphis.usda.gov/animal_health/birdbiosecurity/end/. Accessed May 6, 2011.)

Appropriate housing and nutrition of backyard poultry are necessary to prevent overcrowding, stress, and nutritional deficiencies that may predispose birds to illness. County or state agricultural extension offices are often excellent sources of information regarding flock management practices. In addition, owners should be advised to purchase birds only from reputable, disease-free sources. They should prevent contact between poultry and potential disease carriers such as arthropods, rodents, and wild birds.[6–8] Farm equipment should not be shared between separate flocks and, ideally, visitors to the flocks should not be allowed, especially individuals who have contact with other birds.[9,10] Equipment should be appropriately sanitized. Lists of disinfectants and their spectrums of action have been published in detail elsewhere.[2,10] Owners can be referred to the United States Department of Agriculture Animal and Plant Health Inspection Service (USDA-APHIS) website for additional instructions regarding biosecurity in the backyard flock (**Fig. 1**).[9]

Poultry owners should be taught to recognize general signs of illness in birds so that they can effectively isolate, report, and/or seek treatment for sick birds.[9] Furthermore, they should be educated about the risks of asymptomatic carriers of disease and be knowledgeable of the fact that seemingly healthy birds can transmit zoonotic diseases. Partly because there is a plethora of medical products available over-the-counter to owners, they should be educated about the value of appropriately diagnosing and treating a disease in consultation with a veterinarian. In addition, instruction can be provided regarding the limited number of drugs that are approved for use in poultry, as well as the legal and ethical implications of extra-label use of drugs in backyard flocks. Appropriate vaccination can be an integral part of disease prevention and outbreak control. Education regarding the relative risks of infection and the proper use of vaccines should be presented to the owner. Due to the time, labor, and financial commitments that are involved in treating an infectious disease outbreak in a flock, the value of a diagnostic necropsy should not be overlooked.

In order to decrease the risk of zoonotic disease transmission from poultry, practicing good hygiene and employing personal protective measures is imperative. Hand-washing with warm, soapy water after handling birds or their excrement, and not eating or drinking around the flock are recommended.[11,12] It is also advisable to wear personal protective equipment, which includes gloves, dedicated clothing and footwear, and airway protection (mask, respirator, etc) when working in close proximity to poultry or their aerosolized secretions. In addition, the CDC recommends that children under the age of 5 and immunocompromised people do not have contact with poultry because of the increased susceptibility of these individuals to infectious diseases.[12] Although many backyard flock owners will find these recommendations tedious or impractical, their importance in preventing zoonotic diseases cannot bo ovorstrossod.

BACTERIAL ZOONOSES
Salmonella Species

The gram-negative rod-shaped bacilli of the genus *Salmonella* are currently classified into 2 species, *S enterica* and *S bongori*.[13,14] There are 6 subspecies of *S enterica* and more than 2500 genetically distinct serotypes identified.[14] Although the full classification of a *Salmonella* serovar may be written as *S enteric*, subspecies *enteric*, serovar *enteritidis*, the isolates are frequently referred to simply by their serotype nomenclature (ie, *Salmonella enteritidis*).[15] All *Salmonellae* serovars associated with poultry are of the species *S enteric*, and most are of the *S enterica* subspecies *enteric*.[16,17]

The avian-specific *Salmonella* serotypes that cause pullorum disease and fowl typhoid were formerly known as *Salmonella pullorum* and *Salmonella gallinarum*, respectively. However, recent reclassification may designate them as *Salmonella gallinarum-pullorum* or simply as *Salmonella gallinarum*.[14,18] These bacteria typically cause septicemic diseases with a very high mortality in chickens and turkeys, and they have only very rarely been isolated from humans.[18] According to a CDC report, *S gallinarum* accounted for only 13 out of a total of 390,767 *Salmonella* isolates obtained from humans between 1996 and 2006.[14] The National Poultry Improvement Plan (NPIP), managed through the USDA-APHIS, was designed in part to control pullorum disease and fowl typhoid, and it has succeeded in eradicating them from commercial poultry flocks in the United States.[18,19]

In contrast, the non-host adapted *Salmonella* serovars, designated as the paratyphoid *Salmonellae*, are a significant public health concern, specifically as food-borne pathogens. Paratyphoid *Salmonellae*, including *S enteritidis* and *S heidelberg*, rarely cause systemic illness in mature poultry. However, morbidity and mortality associated with bacteremia in hatchlings can be high, with clinical signs including profuse diarrhea, lethargy, ruffled feathers, and heat-seeking behavior.[15] More often, these organisms are shed in the feces or transmitted within the eggs of asymptomatic birds. Eggs may become contaminated with *Salmonella* either through direct transmission from a colonized reproductive tract during egg formation or through penetration of the eggshell by fecal bacteria after oviposition.[20] *Salmonella enteritidis* is the most common *Salmonella* serovar linked to egg contamination, and it is estimated that one in 20,000 chicken eggs in the United States is internally contaminated with *S enteritidis*.[21] Through the USDA and the Food and Drug Administration (FDA), compulsory programs are in place for commercial flocks with greater than 3000 laying hens to monitor for *S enteritidis* and assure the quality of the eggs and egg products produced for human consumption.[22] Isolation and identification of *Salmonella* through culture of the feces, eggs, egg products, or affected tissues are required to confirm a diagnosis of infection in poultry.[15]

Human salmonellosis results from the ingestion of contaminated meat, eggs, or egg products, or from direct contact with the animal or its feces. A study conducted by the CDC estimated that 1.4 million human nontyphoidal *Salmonella* infections occur in the United States each year.[23] *Salmonella enteritidis* was the second most common serovar isolated from humans in 2006, comprising 16.6% of the isolates.[14] Human exposure to *Salmonella* may result in disease varying from asymptomatic infection to a self-limiting acute gastroenteritis to bacterial sepsis, sometimes resulting in death in very severe or untreated cases. The more severe cases typically occur in the elderly, infants, and immunocompromised patients, or in individuals that were exposed to a large quantity of bacteria.[24]

Preventing *Salmonella* transmission from backyard poultry to humans can be achieved, in part, by following the recommendations for general flock health and personal protection outlined previously in this article. Due to the high prevalence of salmonellosis in children under the age of 5 years, and the increased potential for *Salmonella* to be shed in feces of young poultry, the CDC makes a specific recommendation against the handling of chicks and ducklings by children.[25] As human salmonellosis is primarily a food-borne zoonosis, guidelines for proper handling and preparation of meat, eggs, and egg products should be followed. Eggs should be collected as soon as possible after laying; cracked and excessively soiled eggs should be discarded; and visible debris on the eggs should be wiped away gently with a clean cloth.[26] A pressure gradient between a warm, freshly laid egg and a cooler environment may promote migration of bacteria through the eggshell. Thus, if the eggs are washed, it should be in water that is 10°F warmer than the egg and they should be dried thoroughly with a clean cloth.[20,26] All eggs and meat products should be refrigerated and prepared according to the FDA safety recommendations.[21,22] Unpasteurized eggs should not be used in recipes such as eggnog and ice cream that would result in the consumption of raw or undercooked eggs.[21]

Other Food-borne Bacteria

Additional enteric bacteria that have a potential for zoonotic transmission from poultry to humans include, but are not limited to, *Campylobacter jejuni*, *Escherichia coli*, *Clostridium perfringens* type A and type C, *Listeria monocytogenes*, *Staphylococcus* spp, *Streptococcus* spp, and *Enterococcus* spp. As with *Salmonella*, human infection with these bacteria can occur via direct animal contact or by ingestion of contaminated poultry products. Human illnesses typically manifest as acute gastroenteritis.[27–34] However, severe complications of campylobacteriosis have been reported to include reactive arthritis, Guillain-Barré syndrome, septic abortion, and death. The use of fluroroquinolones in poultry is currently banned by the FDA in response to emergence of resistance to these antimicrobials in *Campylobacter* strains isolated from both poultry and humans.[27,28] Following the recommendations for improvement of general flock health, good hygiene, and appropriate food preparation previously presented in this article should be sufficient to limit the risk of zoonotic transmission of these bacteria.

Erysipelothrix rhusiopathiae

Erysipelothrix rhusiopathiae is a gram-positive bacillus that causes disease in a variety of species including poultry, and especially in turkeys. Clinical signs of erysipelas in gallinaceous birds and waterfowl include skin discoloration, emaciation, depression, diarrhea, decreased egg production, and death. Male turkeys may develop swollen, cyanotic snoods.[35,36] Although the suspicion of erysipelas can be based on clinical signs and gross necropsy findings consistent with septicemia and hemorrhagic disease, the diagnosis should be confirmed with a positive culture of *E rhusiopathiae* from affected birds. A combination of culture and polymerase chain reaction (PCR) techniques may be useful in identifying *E rhusiopathiae* in avian tissues, particularly those sampled from carrier birds.[35]

Erysipelothrix rhusiopathiae is transmitted to humans via direct contact, usually through broken skin, and infection is most frequently reported in individuals that work closely with animals, such as veterinarians and butchers.[35] Three forms of disease can develop in human erysipelas cases: a localized cutaneous form, a generalized cutaneous form, and a septicemic form that is often associated with endocarditis. Zoonotic transmission can be prevented by wearing gloves and practicing good hygiene, including thorough handwashing.[36]

Chlamydophila psittaci

Chlamydophila psittaci is an obligate, intracellular gram-negative bacterium that has been shown to cause infection in over 400 avian species spanning more than 21 orders. Of the 8 known serovars of *C psittaci*, serovars C, D, and E are commonly associated with poultry species.[37] *Chlamydophila psittaci* is particularly prevalent in turkeys, and serovar D is recognized as being highly virulent in the species, with morbidity rates of 50% to 80% and mortality rates of 10% to 30%.[38,39]

Avian chlamydophilosis can be an acute, chronic or asymptomatic disease. Clinical signs in turkeys infected with a virulent *C psittaci* serovar include cachexia, anorexia, conjunctivitis, sinusitis, respiratory distress, yellow-green gelatinous droppings, and decreased egg production.[37,39] Necropsy findings in these birds are nonspecific and can include air sacculitis, pulmonary congestion, hepatosplenomegaly, pericarditis, myocarditis, peritonitis, vasculitis, nasal adenitis, and inflammatory gonadal disease.[37,39,40] Less virulent infections in turkeys typically result in anorexia and loose green droppings. Chlamydophilosis in ducks and geese can cause trembling, ataxia, conjunctivitis, rhinitis, cachexia, anorexia, and green diarrhea.[37,39] Chickens are relatively resistent to *C psittaci* infections, with most natural infections being asymptomatic. However, clinical cases have been reported in domestic chickens and in farm-raised pheasants, quail, and partridges. The biphasic developmental cycle of chlamydial organisms and the ability of the intracellular component of the infection to survive within cellular inclusions are associated with chronic infections and asymptomatic carrier states.[37,40] In addition, this unique infectious biology can make avian chlamydophilosis challenging to diagnose and effectively treat.

Chlamydophila psittaci is transmitted principally through inhalation of aerosolized feces or respiratory secretions from an infected bird, and secondarily through direct contact and ingestion of contaminated feces. There is evidence of vertical transmission and arthropod-vectored transmission between birds. Zoonotic transmission can also occur through bite wounds or broken skin.[39]

The zoonotic potential of *C psittaci* is well-documented, with 66 cases of human *C psittaci* infection being reported to the CDC between 2005 and 2009.[41] Human infections with *C psittaci* are known as psittacosis, ornithosis, chlamydophilosis, or parrot fever.[13,41] Although the majority of psittacosis cases result from exposure to an infected pet psittacine, contact with poultry species, particularly turkeys, poses a significant risk of zoonotic infection.[38,41,42] Acute clinical psittacosis typically presents with symptoms of headache, chills, malaise, myalgia, photophobia, and cough within 5 to 14 days of exposure. Atypical pneumonia is the most common manifestation of human C psittaci infection, and mortality is extremely rare with appropriate antibiotic therapy.[24,41]

The diagnosis, treatment, and prevention of avian chlamydophilosis and psittacosis have been described in detail in a compendium article published by the National Association of State Public Health Veterinarians.[41] Although the compendium is written with a specific focus on avian chlamydophilosis in psittacine birds, testing principles and prevention strategies can be utilized in other avian species. Application of the various testing procedures—including bacterial culture, PCR, and serology, as well as treatment with chlortetracycline-medicated feed in the commercial poultry flock—has been described elsewhere.[37]

Psittacosis in humans is a Nationally Notifiable Disease, and reporting cases to the state or local public health authorities is required in most areas. Guidelines for reporting avian chlamydophilosis vary by state and local regulations.[41] Nevertheless, the movement of poultry, carcasses, or offal from premises with confirmed chlamydophilosis is forbidden by the USDA-APHIS. There is no restriction on the movement of eggs from these flocks.[37]

Mycobacterium avium subspecies avium

Mycobacteriosis has been reported in almost all orders of birds, and the disease in poultry is most commonly caused by the acid-fast bacilli Mycobacterium avium subspecies avium. Mycobacteria are ubiquitous environmental saprophytes and can survive in the soil for years.[43] The susceptibility of avian species to mycobacteriosis is variable and, of the species commonly kept in backyard flocks, pheasants and waterfowl are reported to be particularly susceptible to infection.[44]

Mycobacteria most frequently affect the gastrointestinal system and liver in birds.[43,45] Clinical signs of avian mycobacteriosis are variable and, in poultry, they can include lethargy, cachexia (despite a good appetite), dull plumage, diarrhea, pale or cyanotic comb and wattle, lameness, hepatomegaly, ascites, and decreased egg production.[43,44] Signs of cutaneous, respiratory, ocular, and neurologic involvement are less commonly reported. Birds may also be asymptomatic carriers of mycobacterium and shed large quantities of the organism through their feces into the environment.[44] Mycobacterium is usually transmitted by the ingestion or inhalation of contaminated water and soil.[45]

Ante-mortem diagnosis of avian mycobacteriosis is challenging and should be based on a variety of tests. Fecal shedding of Mycobacterium in infected birds can be limited and sporadic, and Mycobacterium identified in the feces may only represent non-pathogenic organisms transiting the gastrointestinal tract.[43,44] Thus, a presumptive diagnosis made based on fecal cytology, culture, or PCR should be supported by histopathologic features of mycobacteriosis and demonstration of organisms within biopsied tissue.[43,46] Unlike in psittacine birds, intradermal tuberculin tests and whole-blood agglutination tests have been used to reliably diagnosis mycobacteriosis in domestic poultry.[43,44]

Disseminated human mycobacteriosis due to Mycobacterium avium is most common in individuals with acquired immune deficiency syndrome (AIDS) and typically results in fever, weight loss, and anemia with a heavy mycobacterial infection of the gastrointestinal tract.[46] Although birds with confirmed mycobacteriosis are a potential zoonotic risk to humans, it is thought that most human M avium infections are acquired from environmental sources. Owners should be informed of the risks of owning a bird with mycobacteriosis, and should be educated regarding the necessary steps to try and eradicate this disease from the flock.[13,44]

The treatment of mycobacteriosis in avian patients is controversial and variably successful. It typically involves the long-term, daily administration of a combination of human antituberculous drugs.[46] Due to the expense, impracticality, legality, and ethical implications of using these drug protocols in species that could contribute to the human food supply, treatment of mycobacteriosis in backyard poultry is not recommended. Alternatively, it is advised to depopulate the entire flock and repopulate on uninfected soil with new equipment in order to control mycobacteriosis.[43] If euthanasia of affected birds is not an option, they should be permanently isolated from the flock, and the previously discussed biosecurity and personal protective measures should be implemented on the farm to prevent recontamination of the flock and potential zoonotic transmission.[44]

VIRAL ZOONOSES
Avian Influenza

Avian influenza (AI) virus is an RNA orthomyxovirus. The antigenicity of the surface glycoproteins hemagglutinin (H) and neuraminidase (N) are utilized to subtype AI viruses. Subtypes are described as any combination of one of the 16 known H glycoproteins and one of the 9 known N glycoproteins. Subtypes are further categorized into 2 pathotypes: highly pathogenic avian influenza (HPAI) and low pathogenicity avian influenza (LPAI), based on the severity of the disease that they produce in a given species.[47,48] LPAI viruses can mutate into more highly pathogenic forms, as occurred in a 1983 to 1984 AI outbreak in chicken flocks in Pennsylvania, Virginia, Maryland, and New Jersey.[49] All HPAI subtypes are Notifiable Diseases, whereas only the H5 and H7 subtypes of LPAI are reportable.[47]

Signs of AI in domestic poultry are extremely variable and depend on the pathotype of the virus as well as multiple host characteristics (species, age, concurrent infections, and so forth) and environmental factors. In chickens and turkeys, LPAI typically produces mild to severe respiratory disease, decreased egg production, excessive lacrimation, and general signs of malaise. HPAI in these species can cause depression, anorexia, neurologic and respiratory disease, decreased egg production, edema of the comb and wattle with cyanosis and hemorrhage, and diarrhea (**Fig. 2**).[47,48] Death can occur with or without prior clinical signs. Mortality rates are usually less than 5% with LPAI and can be up to 100% with HPAI in domestic poultry flocks. Definitive diagnosis of AI in birds requires isolation and identification of the virus from infected samples, or detection of viral antigen within those samples by technologies such as PCR and immunoassay. Antemortem diagnosis can be achieved through testing tracheal, oropharyngeal, or cloacal swabs.[47]

Avian influenza virus is shed in the droppings and respiratory secretions of infected birds. Wild aquatic birds, particularly of the orders Anseriformes and Charadriiformes, are natural reservoirs for AI and can act as asymptomatic shedders of the virus. AI virus is transmitted by inhalation of aerosolized infected secretions, ingestion of contaminated feces, contact with contaminated fomites, and consumption of infected carcasses. Most cases of influenza in birds are the result of contact with an infected bird. However, transmission between mammals and birds has been reported with the transfer of H1N1, H1N2, and H3N2 swine-origin influenza viruses from pigs and humans to turkeys.[47,50]

Most human H5N1 HPAI cases have been linked to direct exposure to infected live or dead poultry.[8,47] Person-to-person transmission of H5N1 and H7N7 has been reported, but it is rare and unsustained.[24,51] Signs of AI in humans include conjunctivitis,

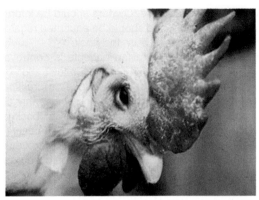

Fig. 2. Swelling of the periorbital region, comb, and wattle in a chicken. These clinical signs can develop with various infectious diseases including avian influenza and Newcastle disease. (*From* United States Department of Agriculture Animal and Plant Health Inspection Service (USDA-APHIS) Biosecurity Guide for Poultry and Bird Owners. Available at: http://www.aphis.usda.gov/animal_health/birdbiosecurity/end/. Accessed May 6, 2011.)

fever, upper respiratory tract infection, cough, and gastrointestinal upset. Humans with LPAI typically exhibit mild signs, but HPAI influenza can progress rapidly to death in humans, with mortality reaching 50% to 60%.[24,47] Humans that are in contact with poultry should employ all the previously discussed hygiene and personal protection methods, including handwashing and wearing masks, to help prevent AI infection.[48]

Co-infection of an individual with 2 influenza subtypes can lead to genetic recombination of the viruses and result in a new strain of virus, with increased infectivity and transmissibility. Although no mammalian vaccination against HPAI virus is commercially available, vaccination with the seasonal human influenza vaccine may decrease the risk of dual infections.[48,52] The influenza vaccine offered in the United States during the 2010 to 2011 influenza season provides protection against the H1N1 and H3N2 influenza A subtypes as well as influenza B.[53] Individuals at increased risk of zoonotic AI infection, including poultry workers and veterinarians that are exposed to birds, are highly encouraged to receive the current influenza virus vaccine.[48,54,55] It has been suggested that those high risk individuals should receive priority access to influenza vaccines and antiviral drugs in the case of an outbreak.[55–58]

The previously discussed flock biosecurity measures are an imperative component to preventing AI outbreaks in domestic poultry. In addition, partly as an effort to prevent HPAI viral strains from entering into the United States, the importation of live poultry, unprocessed poultry products, and hatching eggs from AI-infected countries is restricted by the USDA.[56] In the event of an AI outbreak in domestic poultry, including LPAI H5 and H7 outbreaks, flock depopulation is typically recommended. Government approval is required for the use of AI vaccinations in most countries, and human antiviral drugs are not approved for use in domestic poultry.[47]

Newcastle Disease

Newcastle disease (ND) is caused by a virus of the family Paramyxoviridae, classified as avian paramyxovirus type 1. Strains of ND virus vary significantly in their virulence and can result in subclinical infections or induce respiratory, gastrointestinal, and central nervous system disease in domestic poultry.[59,60] The virus is transmitted

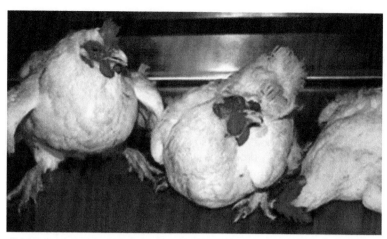

Fig. 3. Chickens exhibiting paresis and torticollis. Infectious diseases that affect the central nervous system, including avian influenza, Newcastle disease, eastern equine encephalitis, western equine encephalitis, and West Nile virus, can cause these clinical signs in poultry. (*From* USDA Food Safety and Inspection Service. Available at: http://www.fsis.usda.gov/fsis_employees/ avian_influenza_training/index.asp. Accessed May 6, 2011.)

through both a fecal-oral route and aerosolization of infected respiratory secretions. Human cases of ND are usually mild and self-limiting. Conjunctivitis is the most common symptom of human ND infection with fever, chills, headache, pharyngitis, decreased appetite, photophobia, and lethargy occurring rarely.[24,59] A live virus vaccine for which there is no withdrawal period is available over-the-counter in the United States. In order to prevent human infection, extreme caution should be exercised, and personal protective equipment should be used when administering this vaccine, especially when it is aerosolized.[61]

Arthropod-borne Viruses

Of the 5 arthropod_vectored viruses known to cause disease in domestic poultry (WNV, EEE, WEE, Highlands J virus, and Israel turkey meningoencephalitis virus), only 3 of these are reportedly pathogenic in humans. WNV, EEE, and WEE all have the potential to cause severe neurologic disease and death in people. In birds, these diseases can be asymptomatic or result in inapparent infection with acute death. If clinical signs develop, they are typically related to central nervous system infection and can include opthisthotonus, torticollis, recumbency, paresis and paralysis, incoordination, and tremors (**Fig. 3**). Of the poultry species, EEE outbreaks are most commonly reported in pheasants, and WNV outbreaks are most commonly reported in geese.[62] Diagnosis of these viral diseases involves virus isolation and identification, demonstration of viral antigen or genomic sequences, and serologic testing.[62,63]

Although mosquitoes and various other arthropods are the primary vectors of these diseases, direct transmission of EEE and WNV by cannibalism and feather-picking has been reported to occur in poultry.[62,64] Zoonotic transmission of WNV through contact with infected animals or their tissues has also been reported.[63] Prevention of infection is typically directed at mosquito control measures—such as eliminating standing water sources and spraying insecticides—and at reducing contact between mosquitoes and vertebrae hosts.[62,63] Remaining indoors during times of high mosquito activity and wearing mosquito repellent may decrease the risk of infection.[63] Vaccination of avian species against the arthropod-vectored viruses has been reported but it is not routinely performed in backyard poultry. To the author's knowledge, avian vaccines for EEE, WEE, and WNV are not commercially available. Extra-label use of equine vaccinations has been performed in birds with relative safety and questionable efficiency.[62,63]

FUNGAL ZOONOSES

Cryptococcus neoformans and *Histoplasma capsulatum* are both fungal organisms that can be passed in avian droppings and survive in contaminated soil. Clinical disease due to *C neoformans* and *H capsulatum* is rarely reported in poultry, and fecal shedding of these organisms is most commonly associated with pigeons.[65] Zoonotic infection typically results from inhalation of organisms. Human infection with *C neoformans* usually produces pulmonary symptoms and meningitis. However, cutaneous lesions are possible if infection is from direct contact through broken skin. Humans with *H capsulatum* infection typically present with fever, chills, headache, nonproductive cough, and chest pain.[24] Aspergillosis is not a zoonotic disease but the *Aspergillus* spp fungal organisms that cause this infection can thrive in decaying organic matter associated with poultry farming.[65] As previously mentioned, appropriate precautions, such as wearing a mask and gloves, should be taken while handling poultry bedding and carcasses to prevent inhalation and contact with infectious agents.

Favus (dermatophytosis primarily caused by *Microsporum gallinae*) is a contagious fungal disease of poultry that is transmissible to humans through direct contact. In both birds and humans, infection results in scaly cutaneous lesions and can be diagnosed through microscopic identification of the organisms on skin scrapings or in tissue samples. Zoonotic infection can be prevented by wearing gloves when handling birds with favus.[65]

PARASITIC ZOONOSES

Fowl mites, including *Ornithonyssus sylviarum* and *Dermanyssus gallinae*, can be transmitted to humans by direct contact. The mites' bites can result in pruritis and erythematous papular eruptions in humans, and definitive diagnosis involves visualization of the mites.[66] Zoonotic transmission can be prevented through eradication of the mites from the poultry flock and wearing protective clothing while handling mite-infested birds.

The protozoan organisms *Toxoplasma gondii* and *Cryptosporidium* spp can cause significant disease in humans, but infection only rarely involves exposure to infected poultry.[67,68] Birds become infected with *T gondii* through the ingestion of infective oocytes, which are passed in the feces of felids. Infections through ingestion of arthropods and earthworms that have ingested oocytes are also possible. Poultry with toxoplasmosis may exhibit symptoms, including anorexia, weight loss, a pale comb, spasms, paralysis, and blindness. However, the majority of infections are inapparent.[67] Although clinical cases of toxoplasmosis are rarely reported in poultry, a variety of studies have shown that viable organisms are present in 27% to 100% of backyard chickens.[69] Zoonotic transmission of *T gondii* from poultry involves the consumption of tissue cysts in undercooked meat. Control methods should be directed at preventing ingestion of feline feces by poultry and destroying tissue cysts through freezing meat or cooking it to an internal temperature of 66°C (150.8°F).[67,69] Of the avian-associated *Cryptosporidium* spp, zoonotic transmission of *Cryptosporidium meleagridis* is of greatest concern.[68,70] *C meleagridis*, which primarily causes diarrheal disease in turkeys and quail, is very closely related to the zoonotic strains of the mammalian *Cryptosporidium parvum,* and zoonotic transmission has been demonstrated in both immunocompromised and immunocompetent humans.[68,71-73] *Cryptosporidium* organisms are transmitted through a fecal-oral route and typically result in gastrointestinal signs such as profuse, watery diarrhea and stomach cramps in humans.[74] As with *T gondii*, the oocytes are extremely resistant in the environment. Prevention of zoonotic transmission should be aimed good hygiene practices, as previously reviewed.[67,68]

Zoonotic infections of poultry parasitic worms are rare. Only the cecal roundworm, *Strongyloides avium,* has been documented to cause human infections. The infective larvae penetrate poultry handlers' skin and can result in transient cutaneous eruptions.[75]

SUMMARY

As the ownership of small backyard poultry flocks becomes more popular and new ordinances are written that allow poultry to be kept in the urban and suburban setting, it may be increasingly necessary for veterinarians to have knowledge of poultry diseases and their associated public health risks. Veterinarians play a key role in prevention, diagnosis, and treatment of zoonotic diseases in their avian patients. In addition, they have an obligation to educate owners about the potential risks of zoonotic transmission and methods of decreasing these risks.

REFERENCES

1. Taylor LH, Latham SM, Woolhouse MEJ. Risk factors for human disease emergence. Phil Trans R Soc Lond B 2001;356:983–9.
2. National Association of State Public Health Veterinarians (NASPHV). Compendium of veterinary standard precautions for zoonotic disease prevention in veterinary personnel. J Am Vet Med Assoc 2010;237(12):1403–22.
3. Centers for Disease Control and Prevention (CDC). Nationally notifiable infectious conditions United States 2011. Available at: http://www.cdc.gov/ncphi/disss/nndss/phs/infdis2011.htm. Accessed January 16, 2011.
4. United States Department of Agriculture Animal and Plant Health Inspection Service (USDA APHIS). Animal health monitoring & surveillance: status of reportable diseases in the United States. Available at: http://www.aphis.usda.gov/vs/nahss/disease_status.htm. Accessed January 16, 2011.
5. Babcock S, Marsh AE, Lin J, et al. Legal implications of zoonoses for clinical veterinarians. J Am Vet Med Assoc 2008;233(10):1556–62.
6. Wales AD, Carrique-Mas JJ, Rankin M, et al. Review of the carriage of zoonotic bacteria by arthropods, with special reference to *Salmonella* in mites, flies, and litter beetles. Zoonoses Public Health 2010;57:299–314.
7. Sanchez S, Hofacre CL, Lee MD, et al. Animal sources of salmonellosis in humans. J Am Vet Med Assoc 2002;221(4):492–497.
8. Dierauf LA, Karesh WB, Ip HS, et al. Avian influenza virus and free-ranging wild birds. J Am Vet Med Assoc 2006;228(12):1877–82.
9. USDA APHIS. Biosecurity. Available at: http://www.aphis.usda.gov/animal_health/birdbiosecurity/biosecurity/. Accessed October 2, 2010.
10. Bermudez AJ, Stewart-Brown B. Disease prevention and diagnosis. In: Saif YM, Fadly AM, Glisson JR, et al, editors. Diseases of poultry. 12th edition. Ames (IA): Blackwell Publishing; 2008. p. 5–42.
11. LeJeune JT, Davis MA. Outbreaks of zoonotic enteric disease associated with animal exhibits. J Amer Vet Med Assoc 2004;224(9):1440–5.

12. CDC. Health risks associated with raising chickens. Available at: http://www.cdc.gov/healthypets/pdf/intown_flocks.pdf. Accessed November 23, 2010.
13. Souza MJ. Bacterial and parasitic zoonoses of exotic pets. Vet Clin North Am Exot Anim Pract 2009;12(3):401–15.
14. CDC. *Salmonella* Surveillance: Annual Summary, 2006. Available at: http://www.cdc.gov/ncidod/dbmd/phlisdata/salmtab/2006/SalmonellaAnnualSummary2006.pdf. Accessed December 14, 2010.
15. Gast RK. Paratyphoid infections. In: Saif YM, Fadly AM, Glisson JR, et al, editors. Diseases of poultry. 12th edition. Ames (IA): Blackwell Publishing; 2008. p. 636–65.
16. Gast RK. Salmonella Infection Introduction. In: Saif YM, Fadly AM, Glisson JR, et al, editors. Diseases of poultry. 12th edition. Ames (IA): Blackwell Publishing; 2008. p. 619.
17. Osman KM, Yousef AMM, Aly MM, et al. *Salmonella* spp. infection in imported 1-day-old chicks, ducklings and turkey poults: a public health risk. Foodborne Pathog Dis 2010;7(4):383–90.
18. Shivaprasad HL, Barrow PA. Pullorum disease and fowl typhoid. In: Saif YM, Fadly AM, Glisson JR, et al, editors. Diseases of poultry. 12th edition. Ames (IA): Blackwell Publishing; 2008. p. 620–36.
19. USDA APHIS. Poultry Disease Information. Available at: http://www.aphis.usda.gov/animal_health/animal_dis_spec/poultry. Accessed December 14, 2010.
20. Gantois I, Ducatelle R, Pasmans F, et al. Mechanisms of egg contamination by *Salmonella enteritidis*. FEMS Microbiol Rev 2009;33:718–38.
21. CDC. *Salmonella* serotype *enteritidis*. Available at: http://www.cdc.gov/nczved/divisions/dfbmd/diseases/salmonella_enteritidis/. Accessed December 14, 2010.
22. U.S. Food and Drug Administration (FDA). FDA improves egg safety. Available at: http://www.fda.gov/ForConsumers/ConsumerUpdates/ucm170640.htm. Accessed December 20, 2010.
23. Voetsch AC, Van Gilder TJ, Angulo FJ, et al. FoodNet estimate of the burden of illness caused by nontyphoidal *Salmonella* infections in the United States. Clin Infect Dis 2004;38(Suppl 3):S127–34.
24. Jorn KS, Thompson KM, Larson JM, et al. Polly can make you sick: pet bird-associated diseases. Cleve Clin J Med 2009;76(4):235–43.
25. CDC. *Salmonella* prevention. Available at: http://www.cdc.gov/salmonella/general/prevention.html. Accessed December 14, 2010.
26. Clauer PJ. Proper handling of eggs: from hen to consumption. Virgina Cooperative Extension. Available at: http://www.pubs.ext.vt.edu/2902/2902-1091/2902-1091.pdf. Accessed December 31, 2010.
27. Altekruse SF, Tollefson LK. Human campylobacteriosis: a challenge for the veterinary profession. J Am Vet Med Assoc 2003;223(4);445–52.
28. Zhang Q. Campylobacteriosis. In: Saif YM, Fadly AM, Glisson JR, et al, editors. Diseases of poultry. 12th edition. Ames (IA): Blackwell Publishing; 2008. p. 675–89.
29. Barnes HJ, Nolan LK, Vaillancourt JP. Colibacilosis. In: Saif YM, Fadly AM, Glisson JR, et al, editors. Diseases of poultry. 12th edition. Ames (IA): Blackwell Publishing; 2008. p. 691–732.
30. Opengart K. Necrotic enteritis. In: Saif YM, Fadly AM, Glisson JR, et al, editors. Diseases of poultry. 12th edition. Ames (IA): Blackwell Publishing; 2008. p. 872–9.
31. Van Immerseel F, De Buck J, Pasmans F, et al. Clostridium perfringens in poultry: an emerging threat for animal and public health. Avian Pathol 2004;33(6):527–49.
32. Barnes HJ, Nolan LK. Other bacterial diseases. In: Saif YM, Fadly AM, Glisson JR, et al, editors. Diseases of poultry. 12th edition. Ames (IA): Blackwell Publishing; 2008. p. 952–70.

33. Andreasen CB. Staphylococcosis. In: Saif YM, Fadly AM, Glisson JR, et al, editors. Diseases of poultry. 12th edition. Ames (IA): Blackwell Publishing; 2008. p. 892–900.
34. Thayer SG, Waltman WD, Wages DP. Streptococcus and enterococcus. In: Saif YM, Fadly AM, Glisson JR, et al, editors. Diseases of poultry. 12th edition. Ames (IA): Blackwell Publishing; 2008. p. 900–8.
35. Bricker JM, Saif YM. Erysipelas. In: Saif YM, Fadly AM, Glisson JR, et al, editors. Diseases of poultry. 12th edition. Ames (IA): Blackwell Publishing; 2008. p. 909–22.
36. Wang Q, Chang BJ, Riley TV. *Erysipelothrix rhusiopathiae*. Vet Microbiol 2010;140: 405–17.
37. Andersen AA, Vanrompay D. Avian chlamydiosis (psittacosis, ornithosis). In: Saif YM, Fadly AM, Glisson JR, et al, editors. Diseases of poultry. 12th edition. Ames (IA): Blackwell Publishing; 2008. p. 971–86.
38. Dickx V, Geens T, Deschuyffeleer T, et al. *Chlamydophila psittaci* zoonotic risk assessment in a chicken and turkey slaughterhouse. J Clin Microbiol 2010;48(9): 3244–50.
39. Longbottom D, Coulter LJ. Animal chlamydioses and zoonotic implications. J Comp Path 2003;128:217–44.
40. Harkinezhad T, Geens T, Vanrompay D. *Chlamydophila psittaci* infections in birds: a review with emphasis on zoonotic consequences. Vet Microbiol 2009;135(1–2): 68–77.
41. NASPHV. Compendium of measures to control *Chlamydophila psittaci* infection among humans (psittacosis) and pet birds (avian chlamydiosis) 2010. Available at: http://nasphv.org/Documents/Psittacosis.pdf. Accessed October 10, 2010.
42. Verminnen K, Duquenne B, De Keukeleire D, et al. Evaluation of a *Chlamydophila psittaci* infection diagnostic platform for zoonotic risk assessment. J Clin Microbiol 2008;46(1):281–5.
43. Fulton RM, Sanchez S. Tuberculosis. In: Saif YM, Fadly AM, Glisson JR, et al, editors. Diseases of poultry. 12th edition. Ames (IA): Blackwell Publishing; 2008. p. 940–51.
44. Tell LA, Woods L, Cromie RL. Mycobacteriosis in birds. Rev Sci Tech 2001;20(1): 180–203.
45. Pollock CG. Implications of mycobacteria in clinical disorders. In: Harrison GJ, Lightfoot TL, editors. Clinical avian medicine. Palm Beach (FL): Spix Publishing, Inc.; 2006. p. 681–90.
46. Lennox AM. Mycobacteriosis in companion psittacine birds: a review. J Avian Med Surg 2007;21(3):181–7.
47. Swayne DE, Halvorson DA. Influenza. In: Saif YM, Fadly AM, Glisson JR, et al, editors. Diseases of poultry. 12th edition. Ames (IA): Blackwell Publishing; 2008. p. 153–84.
48. Philippa JD. Avian influenza. In: Fowler ME, Miller RE, editors. Zoo and Wild Animal Medicine Current Therapy 6. St. Louis: Elsevier; 2008. p. 79–87.
49. McQuiston JH, Garber LP, Porter-Spalding BA, et al. Evaluation of risk factors for the spread of low pathogenicity H7N2 avian influenza virus among commercial poultry farms. J Am Vet Med Assoc 2005;226(5);767–72.
50. Pantin-Jackwood M, Wasilenko JL, Spackman E, et al. Susceptibility of turkeys to pandemic-H1N1 virus by reproductive tract insemination. Virol J 2010;7:27.
51. Kalthoff D, Globig A, Beer M. (Highly pathogenic) avian influenza as a zoonotic agent. Vet Microbiol 2010;140:237–45.
52. FDA. FDA approves first U.S. vaccine for humans against the avian influenza virus H5N1. Available at: http://www.fda.gov/NewsEvents/Newsroom/PressAnnouncements/2007/ucm108892.htm. Accessed February 26, 2011.
53. CDC. Influenza vaccine: what you need to know 2010–2011. Available at: http://www.cdc.gov/vaccines/pubs/vis/downloads/vis-flu.pdf. Accessed February 26, 2011.

54. Cook RA, Karesh WB. Emerging diseases at the interface of people, domestic animals, and wildlife. In: Fowler ME, Miller RE, editors. Zoo and Wild Animal Medicine Current Therapy 6. St. Louis: Elsevier; 2008. p. 55–65.

55. Myers KP, Setterquist SF, Capuano AW, et al. Infection due to 3 avian influenza subtypes in United States veterinarians. Clin Infect Dis 2007;45(1):4–9.

56. MacMahon KL, Delaney LJ, Kullman G, et al. Protecting poultry workers from exposure to avian influenza viruses. Public Health Rep 2008;123:316–22.

57. Kayali G, Ortiz EJ, Chorazy ML, et al. Evidence of previous avian influenza infection among US turkey workers. Zoonoses Public Health 2010;57:265–72.

58. Gray GC, Trampel DW, Roth JA. Pandemic influenza planning: shouldn't swine and poultry workers be included? Vaccine 2007;25:4376–81.

59. Swayne DE, King DJ. Avian influenza and newcastle disease. J Am Vet Med Assoc 2003;222(11);1534–40.

60. Alexander DJ, Senne DA. Newcastle disease. In: Saif YM, Fadly AM, Glisson JR, et al, editors. Diseases of poultry. 12th edition. Ames (IA): Blackwell Publishing; 2008. p. 75–100.

61. Fort Dodge Animal Health. Poulvac®. Available at: http://www.fortdodge.eu/product. asp?name=poulvac-ndw. Accessed January 10, 2011.

62. Guy JS, Malkinson M. Arbovirus. In: Saif YM, Fadly AM, Glisson JR, et al, editors. Diseases of poultry. 12th edition. Ames (IA): Blackwell Publishing; 2008. p. 414–26.

63. Travis D. West nile virus in birds and mammals. In: Fowler ME, Miller RE, eds. Zoo and Wild Animal Medicine Current Therapy 6. St. Louis: Elsevier; 2008. p. 2–9.

64. Banet-Noach C, Simanov L, Malkinson M. Direct (non-vector) transmission of West Nile virus in geese. Avian Pathol 2003;32(5):489–94.

65. Charlton BR, Chin RP, Barnes HJ. Fungal infections. In: Saif YM, Fadly AM, Glisson JR, et al, editors. Diseases of poultry. 12th edition. Ames (IA): Blackwell Publishing; 2008. p. 989–1008.

66. Orton D, Warren L, Wilkinson J. Avian mite dermatitis. Clin Exp Dermatol 2000;25: 129–31.

67. Bermudez AJ. Miscellaneous and sporadic protozoal infections. In: Saif YM, Fadly AM, Glisson JR, et al, editors. Diseases of poultry. 12th edition. Ames (IA): Blackwell Publishing; 2008. p. 1105–17.

68. McDougald LR. Cryptosporidiosis. In: Saif YM, Fadly AM, Glisson JR, et al, editors. Diseases of poultry. 12th edition. Ames (IA): Blackwell Publishing; 2008. p. 1085–91.

69. Dubey JP, Jones JL. *Toxoplasma gondii* infection in humans and animals in the United States. Int J Parasitol 2008;38:1257–78.

70. Ryan U. Cryptosporidium in birds, fish and amphibians. Exp Parasitol 2010;124:113–20.

71. Sréter T, Varga I. Crytosporidiosis in birds—a review. Vet Parasitol 2000;87:261–79.

72. Gatei W, Ashford RW, Beeching NJ, et al. *Cryptosporidium muris* infection in an HIV-infected adult, Kenya. Emerg Infect Dis 2002;8(2):204–6.

73. Akiyoshi DE, Dilo J, Pearson C, et al. Characterization of *Cryptosporidium meleagridis* of human origin passaged through different host species. Infect Immun 2003;71(4): 1828–32.

74. CDC. Parasites-cryptosporidiosis (also known as "crypto"). Available at: http://www. cdc.gov/parasites/crypto/disease.html. Accessed January 14, 2010.

75. Yazwinski TA, Tucker CA. Nematodes and acanthocephalans. In: Saif YM, Fadly AM, Glisson JR, et al, editors. Diseases of poultry. 12th edition. Ames (IA): Blackwell Publishing; 2008. p. 1025–56.

Public Health Concerns Associated with Care of Free-Living Birds

Julia K. Whittington, DVM

KEYWORDS

- Avian • Public health • Zoonosis • Wild bird
- Infectious disease • Biosecurity

INTRODUCTION

Natural and urban habitats, once separate and distinct, are now intermingled in many places through human encroachment of natural environments and the use of areas, once reserved for wildlife, for recreation, habitation, and commercial purposes. New residential developments often promote enjoyment of backyard wildlife and incorporate features such as ponds, gardens, and landscaping that encourage inhabitation by common wildlife species that have adapted to co-mingling with humans. The potential for wildlife populations to serve as reservoirs for zoonotic pathogens has long been recognized. Free-living birds have diverse habitats and ranges, including urban and rural environments, and have the potential for extensive interactions with individuals in their environments. Wild birds are susceptible to select pathogens, some with zoonotic potential, and may be presented for care.

Emerging and reemerging pathogens are on the rise, including the emergence of multidrug-resistant bacteria, and the role of potential reservoirs of pathogens are poorly understood.[1,2] Underlying factors for this increased incidence of emerging diseases may have anthropogenic origins including human encroachment into wildlife habitats and an increasing interest in wildlife species, scientifically and socially.[3] The recognition of the interrelatedness of human and animal health has led to increased surveillance of wild animal populations to assess health and to evaluate implications for human health. The result is better detection of disease and pathogen presence. Public awareness and appreciation of individual wild animals increase the likelihood that animals will be presented for care when found ill in their natural habitats. Wildlife care facilities have seen increasing trends in the instance of infectious diseases, some with zoonotic potential. Maintaining secure and enforceable biosecurity measures that protect patients and veterinary care providers is an important component of facility management. Additionally, knowledge of potential pathogens and their

Department of Veterinary Clinical Medicine, University of Illinois, 1008 West Hazelwood Drive, Urbana, IL 61802, USA
E-mail address: jkwhitti@illinois.edu

Vet Clin Exot Anim 14 (2011) 491-505
doi:10.1016/j.cvex.2011.05.008
1094-9194/11/$ – see front matter © 2011 Elsevier Inc. All rights reserved.

epidemiology in a given population or species will be critical in developing handling and care protocols.

RISK OF INJURY

An inherent risk of occupational injury is present when working with wildlife; the potential for injury to the handler and exposure to infectious disease is always possible. Nondomestic species respond unpredictably when subjected to the stress of captivity and handling. Free-living birds are no exception; some species are capable of causing serious injury to handlers. In this author's experience, wounds secondary to taloning by raptor species are the leading injury of veterinary students working with free-living birds and are exceeded only by rodent bites in the number of reported injuries sustained while working with wildlife. All avian species possess natural defenses and behaviors, most notably biting or tearing with the beak and scratching with clawed toes, that are implemented when attempting to avoid a perceived threat. Even wing flaps can cause blunt force trauma to handlers when avian patients are not securely restrained during handling.

Objective data defining the types or frequency of injury sustained by handlers working with wild birds are scarce.[4] Soft tissue injuries including bruises, abrasions, and small lacerations often require only basic first aid and heal without complication. Injuries to the face and eyes are more serious and can be caused by stabbing or pecking motions of the beak, a behavior commonly observed in sea birds and wading birds. The digits of raptorial species have tendons that allow them to "ratchet" the talons down on unsuspecting prey to prevent escape. Unfortunately, this same mechanism makes it difficult to disengage a raptor's feet from a handler who is being taloned. Often, a second person is needed to aid the injured person by manually opening the flexed digits and extracting the talons from the penetrated tissue. Clear communication between handlers is paramount to safe restraint of free-living birds and care must be taken to secure the head, feet, and wings of the restrained avian patient to prevent injury to both the handler and the patient. Occasionally, surgical repair of wounds incurred while handling wild birds is necessary, and potentially permanent disfigurement or dysfunction can result from tissue damage or associated inflammation. Penetrating wounds often are contaminated, especially if caused through injury from the talons of a raptor. A survey of aerobic bacteria found in the feces of raptor species revealed a wide variety of bacteria that can be surface contaminants on the feet of these birds.[5] *Enterococcus* spp, an opportunistic pathogen causing significant morbidity in humans and animals, were also routinely isolated.[6] Prevention of secondary infection in healing wounds should be of primary concern. Clostridial infections, while not commonly associated with wounds caused by wild birds, are possible and tetanus vaccination is prudent in handlers of wild birds.

BACTERIAL INFECTIOUS DISEASES
Avian Chlamydiosis

Avian chlamydiosis, or ornithosis, is caused by the obligate intracellular bacteria *Chlamydophila psittaci*. *Chlamydophila* spp are distributed worldwide and have a wide range of host species representing 30 orders of birds.[7] Clinical infection associated with pet psittacine birds is well described and presents a significant zoonotic risk for owners of infected parrots. Reports of chlamydiosis in wild birds are most often associated with defined mortality events.[8,9] However, detection of *C. psittaci* has been reported from routine screening of wild birds presented for postmortem evaluation.[8,10] Chlamydiosis-related deaths are most commonly reported in pigeon and dove species, gulls, and passerines. Wild birds often show minimal clinical signs related to chlamydiosis, but those with clinical disease may show signs ranging from conjunctivitis, diarrhea, weakness, ruffled feathers, and ataxia to respiratory distress and death. Chlamydial strains show host specificity resulting in no or mild disease in natural host species of birds and increased pathogenicity in others.[8] A recent report describing C psittaci in raptor species from California reported leukocytosis and splenomegally as consistent findings.[11] Transmission of C psittaci occurs via inhalation or ingestion of respiratory secretions or aerosolized feces from an infected bird.[8] Diagnosis of avian chlamydiosis may require multiple diagnostic testing modalities.[11] Direct detection of the organisms via polymerase chain reaction (PCR) or immunohistochemistry is preferred.[8] Acute and convalescent titers with complement fixation to detect IgG provide supportive evidence of infection if a 4-fold rise in antibody titer is noted.

Human infections caused by C psittaci are most often the result of inhalation of infectious material that has been aerosolized. Fecal material, disturbed during handling, can pose a public health risk. Persons working with infected birds or potentially contaminated environments should wear protective clothing, respiratory protection, and gloves. Signs of infection develop 1 to 2 weeks post exposure in affected people and typically include fever, headache, body aches, and general malaise.[8] Respiratory signs may also be present. The disease is rarely fatal in humans and is responsive to treatment.

Enteropathogens

It has been shown that free-living birds, especially waterfowl, may serve as reservoirs of zoonotic enteric pathogens, most notably Salmonella, Campylobacter, Enterococcus, and Escherichia coli.[12–16] In addition to being able to transmit these enteropathogens to humans, wild birds are susceptible to them as well. Transmitted via the fecal-oral route, exposure occurs through direct contact with infected birds or with material contaminated with the feces of infected birds. Birds that travel migratory routes have the potential to spread enteropathogens long distances and contaminate water sources used by domestic animals and humans.[17]

Salmonella is the most common cause of diarrhea in humans and animals.[18] With worldwide distribution, it has been reported in all vertebrate taxa and appears to show little host specificity. A gram-negative aerobic bacterium, Salmonella has more than 2500 serovars. As an enteric bacterium, Salmonella is often found in waste disposal sites and can be the source of exposure for wildlife scavengers such as gulls and other avian species that use areas associated with humans and their ecology. Wild birds can serve as a reservoir for Salmonella, potentially leading to human and livestock exposure through contaminated drinking water, agricultural crops, or direct contact. Bird feeders help perpetuate bird-to-bird transmission and allow for the development of carrier states. Salmonella, if present, is not consistently shed from the gastrointestinal tract of subclinically affected birds and so may not be detected in populations of wild birds.[19] Reported isolation of Salmonella from feces or cloacal swabs of raptors in the United States ranges from 25% of free-living raptors[20] to 8% of raptor species maintained in captivity.[5] Similar data were found for raptors sampled in Spain.[21] Clinical manifestation of salmonellosis in wild birds includes asymptomatic carrier states, enteritis, septicemia, polyarthritis, osteomyelitis, and death. Outbreaks in wild bird populations are sporadic. Salmonella typhimurium isolated from wild passerines and gulls in the United Kingdom were genetically closely related but distinct from those known to have caused outbreaks in humans or livestock, lending evidence of host adaptation.[22] Care providers of wild birds presented for treatment may be unaware of their risk of exposure and possible infection.

Enterococci are gram-positive facultative anaerobic bacteria that are ubiquitous as commensal organisms of the gastrointestinal tract of vertebrates. Often implicated in nosocomial infections, these opportunistic pathogens are associated with significant morbidity and mortality of humans and animals.[23] *Enterococcus faecalis* is responsible for the majority of human enterococcal infections and was consistently isolated from cloacal swabs of raptor species in one study, with a prevalence approaching 80%.[6] Of added concern is the fact that some of the *Enterococcus* isolates retrieved from wild birds demonstrated a variety of antimicrobial resistance patterns, including intermediate vancomycin susceptibility.[6,24]

Avian Tuberculosis

Avian tuberculosis, a cosmopolitan disease affecting wild and captive birds alike, has recently become an important public health concern. *Mycobacterium avium*, often referred to as *M avium-intracellulare* complex (MAC), is most frequently implicated as the cause of avian tuberculosis. Other mycobacteria causing mycobacteriosis in birds include *M genavense, M bovis, M tuberculosis, M intracellulare, M fortuitum, M nonchromogenicum, M chelonae,* and *M gordonae*.[25,26] Mycobacteria are intracellular, gram-positive rod-shaped bacteria possessing a waxy cell wall, rendering it resistant to destruction and allowing it to persist for extended periods of time in the environment. Avian tuberculosis has a high prevalence in wild bird populations; wild birds most likely serve as a reservoir for *M avium* subsp *avium*, the most common isolate from wild birds and the second most common mycobacterial species infecting both animals and humans.[25] Transmission is through direct contact with infected birds or by indirect transmission through exposure to contaminated soil or water. An evaluation of soil transmission of *M avium* subsp *avium* in a zoological collection demonstrated a 70% infection rate from soil to naive birds and persistence of the bacteria in the soil for longer than 4 years.[26]

Birds with avian tuberculosis have evidence of chronic disease as indicated by poor body condition and poor feather condition. Anorexia, lethargy, weakness, diarrhea, and coelomic distension are often noted. Detection of small, acid-fast, rod-shaped bacteria from feces or cytological samples from affected birds offers a presumptive ante-mortem diagnosis. Ziehl-Neelsen acid-fast stain uses detergents to remove the bacteria's cell wall, allowing for stain uptake, which does not occur with traditional gram or Wright's stain protocols (**Fig. 1**).

The disease is most often fatal after a protracted illness of weeks to months. A postmortem diagnosis of avian tuberculosis should be strongly suspected for birds demonstrating granulomatous lesions on the serosal surface of the intestines or embedded in the parenchyma of affected organs, including the liver and spleen.[25] Bone marrow and respiratory tissue can also be affected depending on the route of transmission but are less often involved in mycobacterial infections of wild bird species. Definitive diagnosis is dependent on detection of mycobacteria in blood or tissues. Culture of the etiologic agent is considered the gold standard for definitive diagnosis, but positive cultures are dependent on multiple factors, including type of media, temperature and oxygen requirements of the species, and time. Some evidence suggests that PCR using 16S rRNA gene primers is useful for detecting *M avium* and is more sensitive than cultures in confirming avian tuberculosis.[26]

Mycobacteriosis in humans is associated with lymphadenitis, and mycobacteriosis associated with *M avium* has seen a surge in incidence since the 1980s due to the increase in human patients with human immunodeficiency virus infection and acquired immunodeficiency syndrome (AIDS).[25] *M avium* subsp *avium* has also been the cause of mycobacteriosis in persons with other immunocompromising conditions.

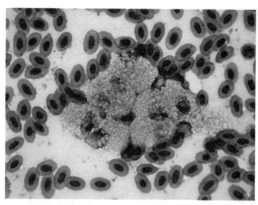

Fig. 1. Fine needle aspirate cytology of liver prepared with Wright-Giemsa stain (original magnification ×1000). An abundance of negative-staining rods are present in the cytoplasm of macrophages.

Human-to-human transmission of *M avium* subsp *avium* has not been reported, making direct contact with infected birds or environmental contamination the likely source of infection in susceptible people. Direct transmission from wild birds to humans is presumed to be possible but data are lacking. Serious consideration should be taken by persons at risk when determining the prudence of working with wild birds that may be carriers of mycobacteria. Avian tuberculosis is sporadic in wild bird populations, and affected individuals may go undetected but still present a public health risk to persons working with the bird. Species that live in close proximity to domestic animals, such as sparrows, starlings, crows, and gulls, are most commonly affected by *M avium*.[27] Puncture wounds infected with mycobacteria are also seen in raptorial species that become infected while grappling with prey or conspecifics on contaminated ground soil. Game birds, cranes, raptors, and waterfowl maintained in captivity are commonly infected, especially when the disease becomes well established with soil and water contamination. Treatment of avian tuberculosis is controversial and is generally not pursued in free-living birds. Infected individuals should be humanely euthanized and contaminated enclosures disinfected. Complete decontamination of natural substrates and water enclosures may be impractical.

VIRAL INFECTIOUS DISEASES
Avian Influenza

Influenza viruses are in the virus family Orthomyxoviridae and are classified as influenza A, B, and C. Influenza A viruses are responsible for most influenza outbreaks and each animal species has its own influenza A viruses.[28] Influenza A viruses are further classified by subtypes based on their surface proteins: hemagglutinin (H) and neuraminidase (N).[29] Hemagglutinin allows the virus to bind to the host cell, causing infection, and neuraminidase is responsible for the release of virus particles from the host cell into the body. There are 16 different types of hemagglutinin and 9 types of neuraminidase. Influenza A viruses are identified by their surface protein type (H1, H2, H3, etc, and N1, N2, N3, etc). Antibodies that the host animal makes to fight influenza infection target these specific proteins; cross-immunity to different proteins does not occur. Influenza A subtypes differ in their species distribution and in the severity of disease produced.[29] Most influenza viruses are highly adapted to a single species or type of animal; however, avian and swine influenza viruses commonly affect other species, including humans. To date, all highly pathogenic avian strains have been H5 and H7, whereas human epidemics have been caused by strains H1, H2, H3, H5, N1, and N2.[30] Influenza viruses are highly adaptable and undergo frequent mutations. These mutations may be small point mutations resulting from antigenic drift that accumulate with time to help the virus avoid the host immune response. Large changes in the viral genome occur when reassortment of large gene segments between viral strains infecting a single host cell results in the formation of a new viral strain. This process, antigenic shift, may produce a viral strain with increased pathogenicity, capable of inducing disease in species that previously demonstrated immunity. The potential for the development of an influenza strain capable of infecting both humans and animals is amplified when a nonhuman host, or mixing vessel, is infected with 2 different viruses.[28] An average of 5% to 20% of the population of the United States gets the seasonal flu annually; greater than 200,000 people are hospitalized for flu-related illness with 4,000 to 49,000 flu-related deaths.[31]

Avian influenza (AI) is a type A influenza virus that has adapted to birds. All avian species are susceptible but domestic poultry tend to be highly sensitive to AI.[29] Two forms of AI are seen: low pathogenic form and highly pathogenic form. The low pathogenic form (LPAI) is found in the United States and worldwide, with affected birds showing no clinical signs or mild disease including slight respiratory signs, ruffled feathers, and reduced egg production. Free-ranging waterfowl serve as a reservoir for LPAI and shed the virus in their excrement.[29] This is a potential source of exposure for birds in backyard flocks or bird markets where LPAI circulates and can mutate into the highly pathogenic form. This mutation occurs at the H protein, which allows for a greater number of protein cleavage sites.[30] Subsequently, more tissue types are infected, resulting in increased morbidity to the host animal. Highly pathogenic AI (HPAI) was first identified in 1878 in Italy. Birds infected with HPAI show sudden onset of severe disease including respiratory signs and massive internal hemorrhage, with virus isolated from multiple organs and tissues. HPAI spreads rapidly and has a high mortality rate in susceptible flocks, which may reach 100% within 24 hours of onset of clinical signs. In areas of the world where HPAI epidemics have occurred in domestic flocks, cases of mortality in wild birds have also been noted. There is still considerable discussion regarding the source of HPAI in wild birds, with some experts suggesting mutation in wild bird populations from LPAI to HPAI and others proposing that HPAI in domestic flocks re-adapts to wild birds.[32] Wild birds infected with HPAI succumb quickly and do not become long-term asymptomatic carriers but can serve to distribute the virus locally in the environment, thereby exposing other birds. AI is transmitted between birds via respiratory droplets and via the fecal-oral route. The virus has also been isolated from feathers of infected birds.[33] AI virus can survive up to 35 days in fecal material at low temperatures and up to 6 days at warmer temperatures and has been isolated from water sources inhabited by free-living waterfowl.[34] Human handlers of wild birds can be a source of vector transmission for AI if virus-laden fecal material contaminates instruments or clothing and footwear of persons working with susceptible birds.[32]

AI is primarily a disease of birds. Since 1997, HPAI H5N1 Asia has caused the death of millions of birds and has resulted in hundreds of human cases, over half of which were fatal, throughout Southeast Asia, Europe, the Middle East, and Africa.[30] However, few cases were associated with transmission from free-living birds and the affected persons were suspected of extensive handling of an infected swan carcass.[35] Despite the fact that HPAI is not an eminent disease in the United States now, it is prudent to develop protocols and personnel safety plans for dealing with any infectious disease outbreak.

Diagnostic testing for HPAI can be performed on live or dead birds. Throat and fecal swabs from wild birds should be placed in sealed sample tubes and submitted to a US Department of Agriculture–approved laboratory for AI screening.[36]

West Nile Virus and Other Arboviruses

Arthropod-borne viruses (arboviruses) are composed of viruses from 12 different families and are transmitted by arthropod vectors.[37] The most common arthropod vector of arboviruses in North America is the mosquito, which transmits the virus after taking a blood meal from an infected host and injecting it into a susceptible individual. Most clinical cases of arboviral infections occur in warm, wet seasons, as this correlates with increased activity of arthropods. Arboviruses are found worldwide and have existed for centuries. Often the animal carriers of the virus do not demonstrate clinical signs of illness, resulting in persistence of the virus in the host population. Wild birds are host to more than 70 arboviruses, most notably those from the viral families Flaviviridae and Togaviridae.[37] Passerines, including house finches (Carpodacus mexicanus), house sparrows (Passer domesticus), American robins (Turdus migratorius), blackbirds, and mourning doves (Zenaidura macroura), among others, are believed to be the primary avian hosts for arboviruses.[37,38]

West Nile virus (WNV), an arthropod-borne flavivirus, emerged as a pathogen in the United States during late summer of 1999.[39] Suspected of originating from endemic areas abroad, the virus has caused significant mortality in birds, humans, and horses. Three hundred twenty-six bird species have been affected by WNV in the United States from 1999 to the present.[40] Members of the Corvidae, Accipitridae, and Strigidae families are particularly susceptible.[37] Thirty-nine states, plus the District of Columbia, reported human cases of WNV in 2010 totaling 981 cases with 45 related deaths.[41] St. Louis encephalitis (SLE) virus is another flavivirus found regionally in North American passerine species, causing significant disease in humans. Unlike WNV, SLE is not a significant pathogen for horses.[37]

Eastern equine encephalitis (EEE) and Western equine encephalitis (WEE) are in the Togaviridae family and are endemic in North America. EEE and WEE have wild bird hosts that serve as reservoirs for the viruses. WEE circulates throughout the western United States and western provinces of Canada and EEE is endemic to eastern North America, the Caribbean islands, Central America, and regionally in South America.[37] The severity of infection in wild bird species varies widely; however, most infections are subclinical in birds living in an area where the virus is endemic.[42] Humans and horses are accidental hosts, and infection rates correlate with levels of circulating virus in bird populations. EEE infections are less common than WEE infections but appear to be more pathogenic for infected humans and horses.[37]

Clinical signs of arboviral infections in birds range from nonexistent or mild to severe and are associated with encephalitis and enteritis. Nonspecific signs include lethargy, cachexia, anorexia, and obtunded mentation (**Fig. 2**). Neurologic signs, including torticollis, opisthotonus, ataxia, paresis, nystagmus, and seizures, may be present upon admission or may develop as the disease progresses (**Fig. 3**). Wild birds that develop severe neurologic disease have high mortality rates. While a presumptive diagnosis of encephalitis secondary to an arboviral infection may be made based on signalment, clinical presentation, hematology, and epidemiology, other differential diagnoses are possible. Serology may give supportive evidence for an antemortem diagnosis but is not diagnostic of active infection. IgM antibody levels are more specific than levels of IgG antibodies but serologic tests are not highly specific for closely related viruses.[37] Serological response secondary to vaccination is highly dependent on species and vaccine used.[38,43–45] Arbovirus-associated viremia in

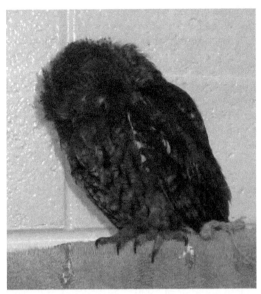

Fig. 2. Eastern screech owl (*Otus asio*) demonstrating clinical signs of lethargy, ruffled feathers, and obtunded mentation, often indicative of systemic infection such as West Nile virus.

birds has a short duration, 1 to 7 days, which precedes clinical signs, making viral isolation unlikely in wild birds presented for clinical care.[37]

Postmortem evaluation of birds suspected of succumbing to WNV may be used to establish a definitive diagnosis. WNV can affect all body systems,[46] and gross lesions

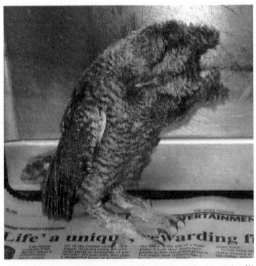

Fig. 3. Juvenile eastern screech owl (*Otus asio*) demonstrating torticollis secondary to West Nile virus infection.

at necropsy are often inconsistent from one case to the next. Findings of hemorrhage in the calvaria, brain or surrounding tissues, gastrointestinal tract, and pancreas are suggestive of disease induced by WNV.[47] Splenic, cardiac, and renal lesions are also commonly described. Histopathology findings include multifocal hemorrhage in the brain, spinal cord, heart, and internal organs. Encephalitis, meningitis, myocarditis, and endocarditis with lymphoplasmacytic or histiocytic inflammation is often reported.[47,48] Disease confirmation is dependent on viral detection by means of immunohistochemistry (IHC), PCR, or virus isolation.

Humans and horses infected with arboviral infections often remain asymptomatic. Those clinically affected will develop mild to severe signs of encephalomyelitis.[42] Clinical signs develop 4 to 10 days after the susceptible person or animal is bitten by an infected mosquito. The ensuing viremia and encephalitis result in fever, muscle aches, and headache. Severely affected people may experience seizures and coma. In extreme cases, the affected person or animal may die from the infection. Treatment is supportive and recovered individuals may have residual impairment. Recent findings support the possibility of persistent WNV in renal tissue of convalescent humans for up to 7 years post infection and the potential for associated renal pathology.[49] Prevention is the key to protecting animals and humans from arboviral infections. Direct transmission from birds is not a significant risk, but evidence exists of infection in humans secondary to transfusions.[50] Care should be taken to avoid contact between open wounds and contaminated tissue. Measures to reduce the population of arthropod vectors, including ticks and mosquitoes, will help to control transmission potential. Other measures include eliminating or removing receptacles where standing water may accumulate and avoidance of being outdoors during times of heightened arthropod activity such as dawn and dusk. Use of insect repellants will also help reduce insect bites and risk of infection.

BIOSECURITY OF FACILITIES

Wildlife care facilities have seen an increasing trend in the instances of infectious diseases, some with zoonotic potential. Maintaining secure and enforceable biosecurity measures that protect patients and veterinary care providers is an important component of facility management. Biosecurity refers to steps taken to prevent risk from the natural or intentional exposure of humans, animals, plants, and the environment to disease-causing biological agents. Biosecurity is based on the principles of preparation, prevention, response, and recovery. Basic to any biosecurity protocol are two main tenets: containment and prevention. These are achieved through identification of potential infectious agents, prevention of their introduction into populations or facilities, and control of their transmission through isolation, treatment, quarantine, or removal of infected subjects. Facilities that provide care for wild birds are presented with a unique challenge. Caregivers must protect hospitalized patients and staff from potential infectious disease exposure while providing treatment for injured, ill, or orphaned wild animals that may be the source of exposure.

Minimum standards for biosecurity are available[51,52]; however, individual facilities must undergo their own risk assessment to personalize procedures. It is important to note that no biosecurity measure is 100% effective and each measure, if adhered to, adds layers of protection to the total plan. Modification of the physical design of an environment, although difficult and costly, is the most effective means of biosecurity enforcement as it does not rely on human behavior or compliance.

The potential for transmission of zoonotic diseases between wild and domestic species or humans increases with their proximity and interaction, either direct or indirect. Human traffic and the use of common treatment areas for wild birds and domestic species increase the risk for pathogen dissemination. It is pertinent to note that 75% of emerging infectious diseases have an animal reservoir and can be classified as zoonotic.[53] Wild birds are known to be reservoirs of several diseases defined as emerging, including arboviruses, influenza A, and enteric pathogens.[17] Patient intake and movement are key points of control in regard to biosecurity. Ideally, wild birds should be maintained separately from domestic birds and animals and should be moved directly to a quarantine area within a dedicated clinical space.[51]

Establishment of minimum health screening protocols for wild birds presented for care is essential to identify infected animals and to monitor disease trends. Diagnostic procedures should ideally include physical exam, baseline hematology, fecal evaluation, and survey radiographs. Further testing should be based on individual animal presentation and species. Consideration of diseases endemic to the facilities' region must be taken into account when developing specific screening protocols.[54] Screening does not preclude the need for quarantine, as incubation periods for infectious diseases vary. If an animal dies from a suspected infectious disease, the carcass should be secured in a plastic bag, avoiding contamination of the outside of the bag, and then double bagged. Gloves used to handle potentially infectious carcasses or tissues should be removed inside out and placed in the second bag before it is secured. The carcass can then be disposed of or submitted for testing. Postmortem examinations should be performed on all free-living birds suspected of infectious disease that are euthanized or die. Proper collection and evaluation of specific tissues will facilitate definitive diagnosis.[55] Medical records for patients should include information such as the age, sex, and species of the animal, as well as the location from which the animal originated, to facilitate disease monitoring.[51]

Isolation is a critical aspect of biosecurity that can both prevent and contain the spread of infectious diseases in facilities providing care to free-living birds. To protect hospitalized patients, birds suspected of infectious disease must be placed in an isolation room with appropriate signage. Equipment and personal protective equipment (PPE) should be exclusive to this area. Ideally, isolation rooms have negative air pressure in relation to the adjacent rooms and should exhaust air directly outside or have the air recirculated using a high efficiency particulate air (HEPA) filter.[56] If a true isolation area is not available, an exam room dedicated to treating infectious birds is preferred. Although not ideal, housing avian patients suspected of infectious disease in mammal wards and infectious mammals in bird wards partially reduces risk of ready transmission between similar species. The purpose of quarantine is to segregate an animal that may be incubating a disease from the main population while monitoring it for signs of clinical disease. Clinical signs of infectious disease are often vague and nonspecific. All animals should be considered potentially infectious and placed in quarantine before being grouped with other patients.

Disinfectants effective against a broad range of pathogens are ideal for facilities housing wild birds. Frequent, routine cleaning and removal of gross contamination, regardless of the disinfectant used, are essential for optimal sanitation. AI virus, an enveloped RNA virus, can be inactivated by all major classes of disinfectants. Disinfectant footbaths and footpads, using peroxygen-based disinfectant, have been shown to reduce bacterial numbers on footwear.[57] Both mechanical removal of organic debris and the antimicrobial activity of the disinfectant help achieve this effect. Adhesive mats offer an alternative and remove contaminants through their adhesive and antimicrobial properties. These measures do not sterilize footwear and should not be relied upon solely to prevent pathogen transmission. Bioaccumulation will require frequent changes of footwear disinfectants. In wildlife care facilities where prevention and containment are equally important, the use of disposable shoe coverings may be useful. Training of personnel to ensure proper removal and disposal of footwear is essential to avoid hand contact with contaminated shoe covers.

The disposal of medical waste is regulated at the state level by multiple agencies including the U.S. Environmental Protection Agency (EPA), which categorizes medical waste as infectious, hazardous, radioactive, and other. Veterinary hospitals, including wildlife care facilities, most often generate infectious or hazardous waste, including sharps, tissues, contaminated materials, and dead animals. Dedicated biohazard receptacles, including sharps containers, should be made available and used routinely in facilities providing care to wild birds. Soiled laundry may also pose a hazard for exposure to potential pathogens and proper handling is required to minimize the risk of disease transmission. Separate clean and dirty laundry bins should be used and gloves should be worn when handling soiled laundry. Machine washing with standard laundry detergent followed by drying is effective in removing contaminants. Rodents and insects are important vectors for the transmission of many diseases. Effective control of rodents is dependent on limiting access to food and nesting material. Food should be stored in air-tight containers, and access to paper, clutter, or hay should be minimized.

PERSONNEL MANAGEMENT

It is essential that worker education is a priority when developing biosecurity protocols. Occupational health and safety plans, based on identification of facility hazards, should be developed. All personnel must be trained regarding zoonosis awareness, infectious disease prevention, safe animal handling, proper use of PPE, basic first aid, and emergency protocols. Additionally, employees must understand their potential role as disease vectors; to become infected or to infect animals with which they work, including pets. Vaccination against rabies, tetanus, and seasonal influenza are often recommended or required by individual facilities.

No PPE is 100% effective. Protective measures must be augmented with good behavioral practices including appropriate hand washing and proper removal and disposal of PPE.[58] Even if PPE is made available, compliance of persons handling wild birds is a crucial factor in successful biosecurity plans. Hand protection should be appropriate for the activities being performed. Disposable gloves made of lightweight nitrile or vinyl offer protection against infectious diseas, while heavy gloves are more appropriate for protection from injury (**Fig. 4**). Care must be taken to avoid contact between contaminated gloves and mucous membranes or noncontaminated surfaces. Nondisposable PPE must be disinfected before storage or reuse. If possible, protective clothing such as lab coats or smocks should be worn over street clothes. Disposable gowns should be used any time infectious disease is suspected. Foot protection, previously discussed, is important to a comprehensive biosecurity plan. Eye protection in the form of safety glasses or goggles protects eyes and conjunctiva from trauma as well as exposure to potential pathogens. Respirators and face shields are recommended for all persons potentially exposed to air-borne pathogens, and are required for those working with patients suspected of having AI.[59] The National Institute of Occupational Safety and Health has approved, as a minimum standard of respiratory protection against AI, disposable particulate respirators (N95, N99, or N100).[59] These require individual training, fit-testing, and use to ensure effective protection. Surgical face masks do not offer adequate protection against particulate air-borne pathogens.

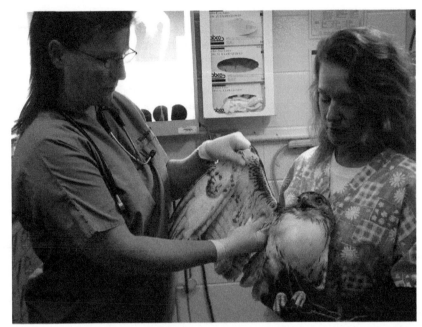

Fig. 4. Examination gloves and protective equipment are important components of effective biosecurity protocols developed to protect care providers of wild birds. Sufficient number of handlers and good communication between handlers will allow for safe handling of wild birds and will prevent injury to personnel during handling.

SUMMARY

Providing care for free-ranging birds can be rewarding and allows for disease monitoring of wild populations. Wildlife care facilities are in a unique position to identify emerging disease through care of wild animal sentinels. Diseases seen in wild birds that are reportable to the World Organization for Animal Health (OIE) include avian chlamydiosis, HPAI, Newcastle disease (neurotropic and viscerotropic strains), and avian mycoplasmosis (*M gallisepticum*). A complete list of reportable diseases is available from the US Department of Agriculture. Recognition of pertinent clinical signs, diagnostic testing, and postmortem diagnosis are essential for detection and management of birds suspected of infectious disease. Preparedness planning for infectious disease outbreaks and developing biosecurity protocols will help ensure the safety of personnel while continuing to care for hospitalized birds. Facility preparedness for infectious disease management will depend on its biosecurity, the monitoring of disease trends in wildlife populations, and open communication with wildlife rehabilitators, wildlife biologists, and government agencies.

REFERENCES

1. Bengis RG, Leighton FA, Fischer JR, et al. The role of wildlife in emerging and re-emerging zoonoses. Rev Sci Tech 2004;23:497–511.
2. Woolhouse MEJ. Population biology of emerging and re-emerging pathogens. Trends Microbiol 2002;10:S3–7.
3. Rhyan JC, Spraker TR. Emergence of diseases from wildlife reservoirs. Vet Pathol 2010;47:34–9.

4. Bovard RS. Injuries to avian researchers at Palmer Station, Antarctica from penguins, giant petrels, and skuas. Wilderness Environ Med 2000;11:94–8.

5. Bangert RL, Ward ACS, Stauber EH, et al. A survey of the aerobic bacteria in the feces of captive raptors. Avian Dis 1988;32:53–62.

6. Marrow J, Whittington JK, Mitchell M, et al. Prevalence and antibiotic-resistance characteristics of *Enterococcus* spp. isolated from free-living and captive raptors in central Illinois. J Wildl Dis 2009;45:302–13.

7. Kaleta EF, Taday EMA. Avian host range of *Chlamydophila* spp. based on isolation, antigen detection and serology. Avian Pathol 2003;32:435–61.

8. Andersen AA, Franson JC. Avian chlamydiosis. In: Thomas NJ, Hunter DB, Atkinson CT, editors. Infectious diseases of wild birds. Ames: Blackwell Publishing; 2007. p. 303–16.

9. Pennycott TW, Dagleish MP, Wood AM. *Chlamydophila psittaci* in wild birds in the UK. Vet Rec 2009;164:157–8.

10. Sharples E, Baines SJ. Prevalence of *Chlamydophila psittaci*-positive cloacal PCR tests in wild avian casualties in the UK. Vet Rec 2009;164:16–7.

11. Hawkins MG. *Chlamydophila psittaci* in wild raptors in northern California: 2000–2009 [abstract 770]. In: Proceedings of the Association of Avian Veterinarians 28th Annual Conference and Expo. San Diego, 2010. p. 349.

12. Dobbin G, Hariharan H, Daoust PY, et al. Bacterial flora of free-living double-crested cormorant (*Phalacrocorax auritus*) chicks on Prince Edward Island, Canada, with reference to enteric bacteria and antibiotic resistance. Comp Immunol Microbiol Infect Dis 2005;28:71–82.

13. Fallacara DM, Monahan CM, Morishita TY, et al. Fecal shedding and antimicrobial susceptibility of selected bacterial pathogens and a survey of intestinal parasites in free-living waterfowl. Avian Dis 2001;45:128–35.

14. Middleton JH, Ambrose A. Enumeration and antibiotic resistance patterns of fecal indicator organisms isolated from migratory Canada geese (*Branta candadensis*). J Wildl Dis 2005;41:334–41.

15. Smith WA, Mazet JAK, Hirsh DC. *Salmonella* in California wildlife species: prevalence in rehabilitation centers and characterization of isolates. J Zoo Wildl Med 2002;33: 228–35.

16. White FH, Forrester DJ. Antimicrobial resistant *Salmonella* spp. isolated from double-crested cormorants (*Phalacrocorax auritus*) and common loons (*Gavia immer*) in Florida. J Wildl Dis 1979;15:235–7.

17. Reed KD, Meece JK, Henkel JS, et al. Birds, migration and emerging zoonoses: West Nile virus, influenza A and enteropathogens. Clin Med Res 2003;1:5–12.

18. Daoust PY, Prescott JF. Salmonellosis. In: Thomas NJ, Hunter DB, Atkinson CT, editors. Infectious diseases of wild birds. Ames: Blackwell Publishing; 2007. p. 270–88.

19. Brittingham MC, Temple SA, Duncan RM. A survey of the prevalence of selected bacteria in wild birds. J Wildl Dis 1988;24:299–307.

20. Lamberski N, Hull AC, Fish AM, et al. A survey of the choanal and cloacal aerobic bacterial flora in free-living and captive red-tailed hawks (*Buteo jamaicensis*) and Cooper's hawks (*Accipiter cooperii*). J Avian Med Surg 2003;17:131–5.

21. Reche MP, Jiménez PA, Alvarez F, et al. Incidence of Salmonellae in captive and wild free-living raptorial birds in central Spain. J Vet Med B 2003;50:42–4.

22. Hughes LA, Shopland S, Wigley P, et al. Characterisation of *Salmonella enterica* serotype Typhimurium isolates from wild birds in northern England from 2005–2006. BMC Vet Res 2008;4:4.

23. Ellerbroek L, Mac KN, Peters J, et al. Hazard potential from antibiotic-resistant commensals like Enterococci. J Vet Med B Infect Dis Vet Public Health 2004;51: 393–9.
24. Fogarty LR, Haack SK, Wolcott MJ, et al. Abundance and characteristics of the recreational water quality indicator bacteria Escherichia coli and enterococci in gull faeces. J Appl Microbiol 2003;94:865–78.
25. Converse KA. Avian tuberculosis. In: Thomas NJ, Hunter DB, Atkinson CT, editors. Infectious diseases of wild birds. Ames: Blackwell Publishing; 2007, p. 289–302.
26. del Pilar Silva A, Leon CI, Guerrero MI, et al. Avian tuberculosis of zoonotic importance at a zoo on the Bogotá Andean plateau (Sabana), Columbia. Can Vet J 2009;50: 841–5.
27. Friend M, Franson JC. Tuberculosis. In: Field manual of wildlife diseases. Madison (WI): U.S. Geological Survey; 1999. p. 93–8.
28. Ritchie BW. Orthomyxoviridae. In: Avian viruses; function and control. Lake Worth (FL): Wingers Publishing, Inc; 1995. p. 351–64.
29. Stallknecht DE, Nagy E, Hunter DB, et al. Avian influenza. In: Thomas NJ, Hunter DB, Atkinson CT, editors. Infectious diseases of wild birds. Ames: Blackwell Publishing; 2007. p. 108–30.
30. Kalthoff D, Globig A, Beer M. (Highly pathogenic) avian influenza as a zoonotic agent. Vet Microbiol 2010;140:237–45.
31. Thompson MG, Shay DK, Zhou H, et al. Estimates of deaths associated with seasonal influenza – United States, 1976–2007. Morb Mortal Wkly Rep 2010;59:1057–62.
32. Causey D, Edwards SV. Ecology of avian influenza in birds. J Infect Dis 2008;197: S29–33.
33. Yamamoto Y, Nakamura K, Yamada M, et al. Zoonotic risk for influenza A (H5N1) infection in wild swan feathers. J Vet Med Sci 2009;71:1549–51.
34. Webster RG, Bean WJ, Gorman OT, et al. Evolution and ecology of influenza A viruses. Microbiol Rev 1992;56:152–79.
35. Gilsdorf A, Boxall N, Gasimov V, et al. Two clusters of human infection with influenza A/H5N1 virus in the Republic of Azerbaijan, February-March 2006. Euro Surveill 2006;11:122–6.
36. Avian influenza diagnostics and testing. United States Department of Agriculture Animal and Plant Health Inspection Service. 2008. Available at: www.aphis.usda.gov/publications/animal_health/content/printable_version/fs_AI_diagnostics&testing.pdf. Accessed February, 2010.
37. McLean RG, Ubico SR. Arboviruses in birds. In: Thomas NJ, Hunter DB, Atkinson CT, editors. Infectious diseases of wild birds. Ames: Blackwell Publishing; 2007. p. 17–62.
38. Kilpatrick AM, Dupuis AP, Chang GJ, et al. DNA vaccination of American robins (Turdus migratorius) against West Nile virus. Vector Borne Zoonotic Dis 2010;10: 377–80.
39. Lanciotti RS, Roehrig JT, Deubel V, et al. Origin of the West Nile virus responsible for an outbreak of encephalitis in the northeastern United States. Science 1999;286: 2333–7.
40. West Nile Virus Vertebrate Ecology. Centers for Disease Control and Prevention. Available at: www.cdc.gov/ncidod/dvbid/westnile/birdspecies.htm. Accessed February, 2010.
41. West Nile Virus Statistics, Surveillance, and Control. Centers for Disease Control and Prevention. Available at: www.cdc.gov/ncidod/dvbid/westnile/surv&controlCase Count10_detailed.htm. Accessed February, 2010.
42. Ritchie BW. Togaviridae. In: Avian viruses; function and control. Lake Worth (FL): Wingers Publishing, Inc; 1995. p. 379–412.

43. Johnson S. Avian titer development against West Nile virus after extralabel use of equine vaccine. J Zoo Wildl Med 2005;36:257–64.
44. Nusbaum KE, Wright JC, Johnston WB, et al. Absence of humoral response in flamingos and red-tailed hawks to experimental vaccination with a killed West Nile virus vaccine. Avian Dis 2003;47:750–2.
45. Olsen GH, Miller KJ, Docherty DE, et al. Pathogenicity of West Nile virus and response to vaccination in sandhill cranes (*Grus Canadensis*) using a killed vaccine. J Zoo Wildl Med 2009;40:263–71.
46. Steele KE, Linn MJ, Schoepp RJ, et al. Pathology of fatal West Nile virus infections in native and exotic birds during the 1999 outbreak in New York City, New York. Vet Pathol 2000;37:208–24.
47. Phalen DN, Dahlhausen B. West Nile virus. Sem Avian Exot Pet Med 2004;13:67–78.
48. Whittington JK, Dietchel SJ, Pinkerton ME. Necropsy findings in wild birds affected with West Nile virus. In: Proceedings of the Association of Avian Veterinarians 26th Annual Conference and Expo. Monterey: 2005. p. 363-6.
49. Murray K, Walker C, Herrington E, et al. Persistent infection with West Nile virus years after initial infection. J Inf Dis 2010;201:2–4.
50. Petersen LR, Busch MP. Transfusion-transmitted arboviruses. Vox Sang 2010;98: 495–503.
51. Miller E, editor. Minimum standards for wildlife rehabilitation. 3rd edition. St. Cloud (MN): National Wildlife Rehabilitators Association; 2000.
52. Sleeman JM, Clark EE. Clinical wildlife medicine: a new paradigm for a new century. J Avian Med Surg 2003;17:33–7.
53. Brown C. Emerging zoonoses and pathogens of public health significance—an overview. Rev Sci Tech 2004;23:435–42.
54. Friend M, Franson JC. General field procedures. In: Field manual of wildlife diseases. Madison (WI): U.S. Geological Survey; 1999. p. 2–71.
55. van Riper C, van Riper SG. A necropsy procedure for sampling disease in wild birds. Condor 1980;82:85–98.
56. Sehulster L, Chinn RYM. Guidelines for environmental infection control in health-care facilities: recommendations of CDC and the Healthcare Infection Control Practices Advisory Committee (HICPAC). Morb Mortal Wkly Rep 2003;52:1–42.
57. Dunowska M, Morley PS, Patterson G, et al. Evaluation of the efficacy of a peroxygen disinfectant-filled footmat for reduction of bacterial load on footwear in a large animal hospital setting. J Am Vet Med Assoc 2006;228:1935–9.
58. Olsen RJ, Lynch P, Coyle MB, et al. Examination gloves as barriers to hand contamination in clinical practice. J Am Med Assoc 1993;2:350–3.
59. Occupational Health and Safety Administration. OSHA guidance update on protecting employees from avian flu (avian influenza) viruses. 2006. Available at: www.osha.gov/OshDoc/data_AvianFlu/avian_flu_guidance_english.pdf. Accessed February, 2010.

Rabies Epidemiology, Risk Assessment, and Pre- and Post Exposure Vaccination

Alice L. Green, MS, DVM[a],*, L. Rand Carpenter, DVM[b],
John R. Dunn, DVM, PhD[b]

KEYWORDS

- Rabies • Vector • Exposure assessment • Vaccination
- Prophylaxis • Risk

VIRUS

Rabies viruses belong to the genus Lyssavirus in the family Rhabdoviridae.[1] The root of the genus name is attributed to the Greek goddess Lyssa, the spirit of rage, frenzy, madness, and rabies[2]; the word rabies itself is derived from the Latin term for madness and raving.[3]

There are over 100 viruses in the family Rhabdoviridae,[2] including vesicular stomatitis and bovine ephemeral fever. Rhabdoviridae are enveloped, single-stranded RNA viruses with a characteristic bullet shape. There are 6 known species of Lyssavirus. Rabies virus is the only one of these endemic to the United States, but all are capable of causing viral encephalitis or rabies-like disease in humans and other mammals.[2]

Variants

Variants of rabies virus in terrestrial animal reservoirs are characteristically host-adapted and limited to a single species in a defined geographic area. However, extension or "spill-over" to other species occurs commonly. In North America, fox variants are maintained in the arctic fox population in Alaska and in limited populations of gray foxes in Arizona and Texas. Raccoon rabies variant is endemic along the eastern seaboard from Florida to Maine, as well as in Alabama, Ohio, Pennsylvania, Tennessee, Vermont, and West Virginia. Three variants are maintained in skunks in 3

The authors have no conflicts to disclose.
[a] Public Health and Epidemiology Liaison, Office of Public Health Science, Food Safety and Inspection Service, United States Department of Agriculture, 100 North Sixth Street, Minneapolis, MN 55403, USA
[b] Tennessee Department of Health, Communicable and Environmental Disease Services, 425 5th Avenue North, Nashville, TN 37243, USA
* Corresponding author.
E-mail address: Alice.Green@fsis.usda.gov

Vet Clin Exot Anim 14 (2011) 507–518
doi:10.1016/j.cvex.2011.05.012
1094-9194/11/$ – see front matter © 2011 Published by Elsevier Inc.

distinct geographic areas, California, and the north central, and south central United States.[4] In Puerto Rico, a variant is maintained by mongooses.[5]

Distinct variants are associated with certain bat species. Geographic range-mapping of bat variants is not possible because of the animals' ability to travel great distances. Since rabies reservoir species of bats are found across the continental United States, every state except Hawaii is considered endemic.[6] Although the majority of human rabies cases in the US since the 1950s have resulted from infection with bat-variant strains,[7,8] the prevalence of rabies virus in apparently normal, healthy bats is reported to be less than 2%.[9–13] The prevalence of rabies in bats submitted to state health departments in the US is somewhat higher, ranging from 8% to 12% positive.[14]

Pathogenesis

Many of the molecular details of rabies pathogenesis are not yet understood. Variability may exist depending on the rabies virus variant and species infected. In general, rabies virus is thought to enter motor neurons at the neuromuscular junction. Virus particles are transported in a retrograde direction through the axon of the infected neuron[15] at an estimated 3 mm per hour.[16] The virus replicates in the neuronal cell body.[17] The mechanism of spread across synapses is unknown.[18]

Replication and transcription of rabies virus reportedly occurs in Negri bodies, cytoplasmic inclusions found in infected neurons.[19] Negri bodies are sometimes used as diagnostic markers for rabies virus infection. Rabies virus does not destroy infected cells, so neuronal transport is maintained.[17] Infection also produces minimal amounts of viral components, and these appear to be contained within the nervous system during initial infection, resulting in only a minor humoral immune response.[20]

After infection of the brain, the virus travels to other body tissues by way of sympathetic, parasympathetic, and cranial nerves.[21] Upon entry into the salivary glands, the virus replicates in mucogenic acinar cells and is released into the saliva.[22] Rabies virus infection results in few gross or histopathologic lesions, despite the severe clinical neurological signs of the disease.[21] Hemorrhage and tissue necrosis of the infected brain are not commonly seen.[23]

In 60% or more of human cases, the incubation period is between 20 and 90 days,[24] and rabies develops within 6 months of exposure in 90% of human cases.[25] Extended incubation periods of 5 years or more have been reported.[26] More severe injuries or head injuries are associated with shorter incubation periods, and incubation periods of 5 days have been documented.[27]

Clinical

Similar to viral pathogenesis, variability in clinical signs and progression may be influenced by the rabies virus variant and species infected. Studies of rabies in dogs demonstrated an average incubation period of 3 to 8 weeks, with a range from 10 days to over 8 months.[28] In cats, the average incubation period is 2 months, varying from 2 weeks to several months or longer.[29] Incubation periods in bats range from 3 weeks to more than 209 days.[30] The incubation period in experimentally infected horses in one study was 12 days; death occurred at an average of 6 days after clinical onset.[31] Cattle in an experimental study had an average incubation period of 15 days, with death occurring 4 days after clinical onset; sheep in the study had an average incubation period of 10 days.[32] A single Vietnamese potbellied pig from Maryland had an incubation period of 4.5 months, which was substantially longer than the 17-day incubation reported for a Vietnamese potbellied pig from Massachusetts.[33]

The 2 types of clinical presentation are generally described as encephalitic (furious) and paralytic (dumb). Among lay persons, the furious form of the disease is the expected presentation. However, in the authors' experience with canines infected with north central skunk variant rabies in Tennessee, paralytic rabies is characteristic. Common signs seen by Tennessee veterinarians and pet owners interviewed over a 3-year period included lethargy, weakness, tremors, hydrophobia, anorexia, salivation, dropped jaw, mild fever, and dysphagia. Increased excitability and irritability were also commonly reported. This is consistent with other research suggesting that rabid dogs are more likely to be lethargic and obtunded, while rabid cats are more likely to be aggressive.[34]

In Tennessee in 2010, a pet Vietnamese pot-bellied pig infected with skunk-variant rabies demonstrated signs consistent with spinal cord injury, including sudden-onset bilateral hind-end paresis, as well ileus and urine stasis. Abdominal guarding, anorexia, fever, and vocalization were also present (L.R. Carpenter, personal communication, 2010). Clinical signs in another laboratory-confirmed Vietnamese potbellied pig with raccoon-variant rabies from Maryland included head and face rubbing to such an extent that all hair was rubbed off the pig's head and jaw, followed by lack of appetite and inability to swallow, fever, and spontaneous vocalization several days later.[33]

In experimentally infected horses, muzzle tremors were the first documented clinical sign, followed by pharyngeal spasm or paresis, ataxia, lethargy, and weakness. More than 40% of horses displayed encephalitic signs.[31] In experimentally infected cattle, clinical signs included excessive salivation, bellowing, aggression, increased excitability, and pharyngeal spasm. About 70% of cattle in the study were classified as having encephalitic rabies. In experimentally infected sheep, muzzle and head tremors were seen, as were aggression, increased excitability, locked jaw, excessive salivation, bleating, and recumbency. About 80% of sheep had encephalitic rabies.[32]

Wildlife species, including many exotic species kept as pets, differ in clinical progression relative to domestic animals. Published incubation period data are not available for many exotic species. The period of clinical illness may be prolonged, as is viral shedding prior to onset of clinical signs. For example, clinical illness in rabid skunks ranges from 1 to 18 days.[35] Bats have been documented as transmitting rabies 12 days before the appearance of clinical signs and 24 days before death.[30] Viral shedding prior to onset of clinical signs poses a risk to wildlife and exotics veterinarians as well as others who work with, or come in contact with rabies vector species. It is possible that a person exposed could develop clinical disease before clinical signs appear in the biting animal.[14]

Prevalence and Distribution in US Animals

During 2009, there were 6,690 documented cases of animal rabies in 49 states and Puerto Rico. About 92.5% of cases were in wildlife; 7.5% were in domestic animals. This is a decrease from 2008, during which 6,841 documented cases of animal rabies occurred. Over one-third of animal rabies cases in 2009 were in raccoons (34.8%; 2,327), and about a quarter each were in bats (24.3%; 1,625) and skunks (24.0%; 1,603), respectively. The remainder of cases included foxes (7.5%; 504), cats (4.5%; 300), dogs (1.2%; 81), and cattle (1.1%; 74).[35] States in the northeast and mid-Atlantic accounted for 67.5% of the total rabies cases in raccoons during 2008. Southeastern states including Alabama, Florida, Georgia, North Carolina, South Carolina, and Tennessee reported 31.5% of raccoon cases (**Fig. 1**).[36]

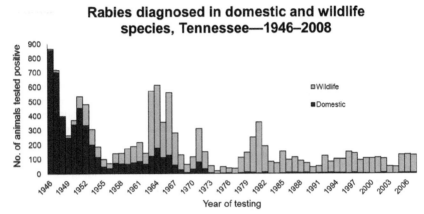

Fig. 1. In Tennessee, as in the United States overall, rabies has transitioned from being primarily a disease of domestic animals to primarily a disease of wildlife.

Rabid bats were reported in all states in the continental US. There were no reports of bat rabies in Alaska, Hawaii, or Puerto Rico in 2009.[36]

Other species of wildlife in which rabies occurred in 2009 included mongooses (34), groundhogs (32), bobcats (30), coyotes (11), fishers (3), white-tailed deer (2), opossums (3), rabbits (2), beavers (2), river otters (2), squirrels (2), muskrat (1), rabbit (1), ringtail (1), wolf (1), and cougar (1). Other domestic animals in which rabies occurred included horses and mules (41), sheep and goats (8), and a ferret (1).[36]

Prevalence and Distribution in Canada and Mexico

Canada documented 145 cases of rabies in domestic and wild animals in 2009; 84% of these were in wild animals. Mexico reported 171 cases of animal rabies; most cases (78.0%) were in cattle.[36]

PREVENTION
Vaccination of Livestock and Pets

All dogs, cats, and ferrets should be vaccinated against rabies. Vaccines should be administered by or under the direct supervision of a veterinarian. One year after initial vaccination, a booster vaccine should be given. After the first booster, the vaccine schedule should depend on the labeled duration of the vaccine[37] and on state or local requirements. Animals with a documented history of vaccination without substantial gaps in vaccination coverage are unlikely to contract rabies even after interaction with rabid animals.[38–40] Post-exposure titers cannot be used as a substitute for booster vaccine.[41–43] Dogs, cats, ferrets, and horses should be currently vaccinated prior to interstate transit according to state requirements and interstate health certificates should document vaccination status. Horses in fairs and other expositions where they might come into contact with the public should be vaccinated.[44] Vaccination of valuable livestock should be considered, particularly in areas where terrestrial rabies is endemic.[37]

IMRAB 3 (Merial, Athens, GA, USA) and Rabvac-3 (Boehringer Ingelheim Vetmedica, Inc, St. Joseph, MO, USA) are killed products used in certain domestic animals. IMRAB 3 is licensed for use in dogs, cats, ferrets, horses, cattle, and sheep. Veterinarians working with exotic animals such as procyonids and exotic felids may wish to consider vaccinating according to ferret recommendations, as advised at one veterinary teaching hospital (M. Souza, personal communication, January 2, 2011). Veterinarians working with llama and alpaca in regions where skunk rabies is endemic may wish to discuss off-label vaccination with camelid owners or other livestock owners. Vaccines recommended at one veterinary teaching hospital for use in camelids include IMRAB 3 or IMRAB Large Animal (currently not available), Defensor 3, Rabdomun, or Prorab-1. All of these vaccines are labeled for cattle or sheep. Recommended dosing and administration for llama and alpaca is the same as for cattle or sheep (R. Callan, personal communication, July 14, 2010).

Use of rabies vaccines in exotic mammals likely reduces, but does not eliminate, the risk of rabies. There are no vaccines approved by the FDA for use in wild or exotic animals, aside from Raboral V-RG used in the USDA's coyote and raccoon vaccination campaigns (Raboral V-RG is not available to private practitioners). Wildlife may be incubating rabies when captured and should be quarantined for 6 months before intermixing with other exotics. When vaccination is performed, only killed vaccine should be used. Modified live vaccines licensed for domestic animals may produce clinical rabies in exotic or wild species. When rabies is suspected in an exotic animal, and a human or domestic animal exposure has occurred, it is recommended to euthanize and test the animal. Observation periods are not appropriate, as duration of viral shedding before clinical onset is unknown.[14,37]

Unvaccinated dogs, cats, ferrets, and livestock with a bite or non-bite exposure from a rabid animal should be euthanized. If this is not acceptable to the owner, the animal should be placed in strict isolation for 6 months so that direct contact with people and other animals does not occur. Rabies vaccine should be administered upon initiation of the quarantine period or one month prior to release.[37]

Another alternative for post-exposure treatment of unvaccinated domestic animals is utilized in some states and is reportedly effective in preventing rabies. The Texas Administrative Code recommends either euthanasia or immediate vaccination of rabies-exposed unvaccinated domestic animals, with booster vaccinations given during the third and eighth weeks of the 90-day isolation period. The protocol can only be utilized in species for which a USDA-licensed vaccine is available.[45]

State or local public health authorities can assist with assessment of animals that are not currently vaccinated but have some history of vaccination. Important factors to consider include vaccination history with number of veterinarian-documented vaccinations given, time since last vaccination, type of exposure, and local rabies epidemiology. If animals exhibit unusual behavior or health problems during quarantine, veterinary and public health consultation is advised. Currently vaccinated dogs, cats, ferrets, and livestock with a rabies exposure should be revaccinated and observed for 45 days.[37]

For further guidance please refer to the National Association of State and Public Health Veterinarians Compendium of Animal Rabies Control (http://www.nasphv.org/Documents/RabiesCompendium.pdf).

Education

Veterinarians in private and public health practice have important roles in rabies prevention and control. Public education about the dangers of handling wildlife can prevent exposures. When exposure occurs, timely risk assessment and post-exposure prophylaxis prevent rabies. Guidance on responsible pet ownership, including the need to keep pets currently vaccinated against rabies and seek timely veterinary care in exposure situations, protects both pets and people. Awareness of the availability of public health guidance is critical for the public and medical professionals. State and local laws requiring vaccination of cats, dogs, and ferrets, and removal of stray animals, are major components of rabies prevention.

Oral Rabies Vaccination of Wildlife

Oral rabies vaccination (ORV) of wildlife has become an important component of rabies management in North America. ORV involves distribution of vaccine-containing baits targeting particular wildlife species to establish population immunity and prevent the spread of disease.[46] ORV has been used with success in Ontario against arctic fox variant rabies in red foxes from 1989–1999.[47,48] Since 1995 an ORV program against gray fox variant rabies has been carried out in west-central Texas.[49] A 1995-2006 ORV program is credited with eliminating canine-variant rabies from coyotes in southern Texas[50,51] resulting in the United States declaration of freedom from canine-variant rabies in 2007.[4]

A priority of the National Rabies Management Program is to prevent the spread of raccoon-variant rabies.[52] Vaccine distribution along the Appalachian Ridge creates a 40–50 km zone of vaccinated raccoons to help prevent the spread of the virus. Starting in 1997, the vaccine distribution zone was expanded to include parts of Ohio, Pennsylvania, West Virginia, Virginia, Tennessee, North Carolina, Georgia, and Alabama. Occasional contingency actions have been needed when positive raccoons are found west of the vaccine border; however, the ORV program has prevented westward spread of the virus among raccoons.[53]

Human Pre-Exposure Vaccination

Pre-exposure prophylaxis should be limited to people with a relatively high risk of exposure, such as veterinarians and other veterinary staff, laboratory workers testing for or experimenting with rabies virus (and husbandry staff caring for any laboratory animals), cavers/spelunkers, and certain international travelers. Three intramuscular injections are required on days 0, 7, and 21 or 28. Booster doses every 2 to 3 years may be recommended depending on titers.[3] Titer measurement every 2 years is advisable; if the titer is less than complete neutralization at 1:5 serum dilution using the rapid fluorescent foci inhibition test (RFFIT), a booster dose of vaccine should be given.[54]

Human Exposure Considerations

Bites from terrestrial animals are high risk and typically obvious rabies exposures; however, nonbite exposure must also be assessed. Nonbite exposure can occur when saliva comes into contact with fresh, open cuts in the skin, or onto mucous membranes. Saliva contact with intact skin and animal handling such as petting or contact with urine, feces, or blood should not be considered exposures. Because bats may bite without leaving an obvious wound, any bat exposure should be assessed with particular care. According to CDC guidelines, finding a bat in the same room with a sleeping person, a young child, or anyone else who might be a poor historian might qualify as an exposure.[54] Additionally, bat rabies variants associated with silver-haired bats and eastern pipistrelles may have a higher likelihood of infection after surface inoculation into the epidermis.[55] As an enveloped virus, rabies is fragile and breaks down readily when exposed to ultraviolet light, sunlight, or dessication.[1] Generally, if saliva from a rabid animal has dried, the virus can be considered noninfectious.[54] Rabies virus remains viable in a carcass for less than 24 hours at 20°C, though it survives longer under refrigeration.[1]

Humans with a possible exposure to a rabies vector species such as a skunk, raccoon, bat, or fox should seek medical care and consult public health authorities.

If available, the animal should be submitted for testing as soon as possible to a state public health laboratory. No observation period exists for wildlife. Post-exposure prophylaxis should be considered but may be delayed if testing is in progress. Circumstances which might prompt initiation of post-exposure prophylaxis while awaiting test results might include a bite exposure to the head or neck. If the animal is not available for testing, or if test results are inconclusive or unsatisfactory, post-exposure treatment should begin as soon as possible.[54]

Humans with a possible rabies exposure from domestic dogs, cats, or ferrets should also seek medical care and consult public health authorities. The dog, cat, or ferret should be observed for ten days according to state and local requirements or tested if not available for observation because of euthanasia or death. Observation is preferable to euthanasia and testing, both for lab resource conservation and animal welfare. Dogs, cats, and ferrets that remain alive and healthy for ten days after a bite would not have been shedding rabies virus in their saliva at the time of the bite.[56] If an animal under observation becomes ill during this time, veterinary evaluation, euthanasia, and rabies testing are recommended. If rabies is confirmed, administration of post-exposure treatment to the exposed person is recommended.

Possible rabies exposures from other wildlife which are not rabies vector species, or from domestic cats, dogs, or ferrets unavailable for observation should be discussed with public health officials at the state or local level. Many states employ designated State Public Health Veterinarians within state health departments to assess and advise regarding rabies risks on a case-by-case basis. Multiple factors must be assessed in addition to the animal species, including whether the interaction was provoked, the appearance and behavior of the animal, and whether rabies is enzootic in the area. Bites that occur while attempting to feed or handle an animal should be considered provoked. Bites from squirrels, hamsters, rats, mice, and other small mammals rarely require postexposure prophylaxis.[54] However, woodchucks and beavers have contracted rabies in raccoon-variant endemic areas.[57]

Post-Exposure Prophylaxis in Humans

After a bite from a rabid animal, wound care is an important part of rabies prevention. Washing the wound with soap and water and when possible irrigation with a virucidal solution such as povidone-iodine are recommended.[58,59] In the United States, human rabies immune globulin (HRIG) from the sera of hyperimmunized donors is available from 2 manufacturers, Bayer (BayRab), and Pasteur Merieux (Imogam Rabies-HT). Post-exposure treatment of people with no previous vaccination for rabies should include both passive antibody and vaccine for both bite and nonbite exposures. If possible, the entire dose of HRIG should be infiltrated around the bite wound. Remaining immune globulin should be given intramuscularly at a site far from that used for vaccine. HRIG is given once at a dose of 20 IU/kg, ideally on the day that post-exposure vaccination begins. If HRIG is not available at that time, it can be given through day 7 of the prophylaxis series.[58]

There are 2 vaccines licensed for human use in the US, human diploid cell vaccine (Imovax), and purified chick embryo cell vaccine (RabAvert).[3] The preferred vaccination site for adults is the deltoid area; for children, the lateral aspect of the thigh is an option as well. The gluteal area should not be used for rabies vaccine because lower neutralizing titers can result.[60] Intramuscular (IM) 1.0 mL doses of vaccine should be given on days 0, 3, 7, and 14, for those who are not immunocompromised; individuals with reduced immunocompetence should receive a fifth dose of vaccine on day 28. CDC published the 4-dose recommendations of the Advisory Committee on Immunization Practices in March 2010; prior to this change, the

5-dose regimen was the standard of care.[61] Package inserts still refer to a 5-dose regimen.

Those who have received pre- or post-exposure vaccine series prior to the exposure in question should not receive HRIG, and only 2 IM doses of vaccine should be given, one on day 0 and one on day 3.[54]

Testing

Rabies testing is performed in laboratories designated by the state or local health department. Direct fluorescent antibody (DFA) staining of brain tissue is the standard for diagnosis, which can be made after detection of rabies in any part of the brain. To rule out rabies, the test must include tissue from at least 2 locations in the brain. Brain stem and cerebellum are preferred. Euthanasia should maintain the structural integrity of the brain; ideally samples should be shipped in a refrigerated state (not frozen) without chemical fixatives.[37] Immunofluorescence testing does not require the presence of viable virus. Viral antigen can be detected for 5 to 7 days at 25°C or for less time at 37°C.[1]

In humans suspected of having rabies, multiple specimens should be collected for antemortem diagnosis in consultation with state public health officials. Testing is conducted by CDC. Specimens include cerebral spinal fluid, serum, saliva, and skin biopsy. A preferred procedure is DFA staining of a skin biopsy from the nape of the neck, above the hairline,[62] as the virus has a tendency to localize in hair follicles. During the first week of symptoms, a single sample has about 50% sensitivity. As time passes, the sensitivity increases.[63] Reverse-transcriptase PCR (RT-PCR) is another diagnostic procedure for use in suspected human rabies.[64] It can be performed on CSF, saliva, or tissue. RT-PCR can be used to determine the species of origin of a particular rabies virus.[65,66] The RFFIT is a serologic test for detecting neutralizing rabies antibody.[67] Fifty percent of untreated patients have detectable antibody by day 8 of clinical illness, and usually 100% by day 15.[68]

Clinical rabies is uniformly fatal, with rare exceptions. Recovery has been documented in only 6 human patients worldwide, five of whom received pre-exposure vaccine.[69,70] In February 2009, the first report of recovery from rabies without intensive care was diagnosed in a 17-year-old girl. She had a prior history of contact with flying bats. Multiple hospitalizations were required but the disease course was shorter and resulted in less severe neurologic problems than were seen in previous known survivors.[71]

In many ways, including educating the public, vaccinating livestock and pets, and observation or timely testing of suspect cases, veterinarians in private practice have an integral role in protection of people and domestic animals against rabies. Rabies should always be considered in the differential diagnosis of a neurologic mammal disease with an unknown vaccination status. Public health veterinarians are available to assist in exposure and risk assessment as well as coordination of animal testing.

REFERENCES

1. Greene CE, Dreesen DW. Rabies. In: Greene CE, editor. Infectious diseases of the dog and cat. 2nd edition. Philadelphia: W.B. Saunders Company; 1998. p. 114–26.
2. Constantine DG. Rabies. In: Wallace RB, Doebbeling BN, editors. Public health and preventive medicine. 14th edition. Stamford (CT): Appleton & Lange; 1998. p. 349–53.
3. Bassin SL, Rupprecht CE, Bleck TP. Rhabdoviruses. In: Mandell GL, Bennett JE, Dolin R, editors. Mandell, Douglas, and Bennett's principles and practice of infectious diseases. 7th edition. Philadelphia: Churchill Livingstone Elsevier; 2010. p. 2249–58.

4. Slate D, Algeo TP, Nelson KM, et al. Oral rabies vaccination in North America: Opportunities, complexities, and challenges. Negl Tropl Dis 2009;3:1–9.
5. Everard CO, Everard JD. Mongoose rabies in the Caribbean. Ann N Y Acad Sci 1992;653:356–66.
6. Blanton JD, Palmer D, Christian KA, et al. Rabies surveillance in the United States during 2007. J Am Vet Med Assoc 2008;233:884–97.
7. Messenger SL, Smith JS, Rupprecht CE. Emerging epidemiology of bat-associated cryptic cases of rabies in humans in the United States. Clin Infect Dis 2002;35:738–47.
8. Noah DL, Drenzek CL, Smith JS, et al. Epidemiology of human rabies in the United States, 1980 to 1996. Ann Intern Med 1998;128:922–30.
9. Venters HD, Hoffert WR, Schatterday JE, et al. Rabies in bats in Florida. Am J Public Health 1954;44:182–5.
10. Girard KF, Hitchcock HB, Edsall G, et al. Rabies in bats in southern New England. N Engl J Med 1965;272:75–80.
11. Trimarchi CV, Debbie JG. Naturally occurring rabies virus and neutralizing antibody in two species of insectivorous bats of New York State. J Wildl Dis 1977;13:366–9.
12. Constantine DG. Health precautions for bat researchers. In: Kunz TH, editor. Ecological and behavioral methods for the study of bats. Washington, DC: Smithsonian Institution Press;1988. p. 491–528.
13. Yancey FD, Raj P, Neill SU, et al. Survey of rabies among free-flying bats from the big bend region of Texas. Occasional Papers, Museum of Texas Tech University 1997; 165:1–5.
14. Constantine DG. Bat rabies and other lyssavirus infections. Reston, VA: U.S. Geological Survey Circular 1329; 2009.
15. Kelly RM, Strick PL. Rabies as a transneuronal tracer of circuits in the central nervous system. J Neurosci Methods 2000;103:63–71.
16. Tsiang H. Evidence for an intraaxonal transport of fixed and street rabies virus. J Neuropathol Exp Neurol 1979;38:286–99.
17. Schnell MJ, McGettigan JP, Wirblich C, et al. The cell biology of rabies virus: using stealth to reach the brain. Nature Reviews 2010;8:51–61.
18. Dietzschold B, Jianwei L, Faber M, et al. Concepts in the pathogenesis of rabies. Future Virol 2008;3:481–90.
19. Lahaye X, Vidy A, Pomier C, et al. Functional characterization of Negri bodies (NBs) in rabies virus infected cells: evidence that NBs are sites of viral transcription and replication. J Virol 2009;83:7948–58.
20. Faber M, Bette M, Preuss MA, et al. Overexpression of the rabies virus glycoprotein results in enhancement of apoptosis and antiviral immune response. J Virol 2002;76: 3374–81.
21. Murphy FA. Rabies pathogenesis. Arch Virol 1977;54:279–97.
22. Balachandran A, Charlton K. Experimental rabies infection of non-nervous tissues in skunks (Mephitis mephitis) and foxes (Vulpes vulpes). Vet Pathol 1994;31:93–102.
23. Jackson AC, Rossiter JP. Apoptosis plays an important role in experimental rabies virus infection. J Virol 1997;71:5603–7.
24. Smith JS, Fishbein DB, Rupprecht CE, et al. Unexplained rabies in three immigrants in the United States: a virological investigation. N Engl J Med 1991;324:205–11.
25. Lakhanpal U, Sharma RC. An epidemiological study of 177 cases of human rabies. Int J Epidemiol 1985;14:614–7.
26. Johnson N, Fooks A, McColl K. Human rabies case with long incubation, Australia. Emerg Infect Dis 2008;14:1950–1.
27. Kureishi A., Xu LZ, Wu H, et al. Rabies in China: recommendations for control. Bull World Health Organ 1992;70:443–50.

28. Tierkel ES. Canine rabies. In: Baer GM, editor. The natural history of rabies. New York: Academic Press; 1975. p. 123–37.
29. Frymus T, Addie D, Belák S, et al. Feline rabies: ABCD guidelines on prevention and management. J Feline Med Surg 2009;11:585–693.
30. Constantine DG. Rabies. In: Hoeprich PD, Jordan MC, Ronald AR, editors. Infectious diseases. 5th edition. Philadelphia: JB Lippincott; 1994. p. 1154–67.
31. Hudson LC, Weinstock D, Jordan T, et al. Clinical presentation of experimentally induced rabies in horses. Zentralbl Veterinarmed B 1996;43:277–85.
32. Hudson LC, Weinstock D, Jordan T, et al. Clinical presentation of experimentally induced rabies in cattle and sheep. Zentralbl Veterinarmed B 1996;43:85–95.
33. DuVernoy TS, Mitchell KC, Myers RA, et al. The first laboratory-confirmed rabid pig in Maryland, 2003. Zoonoses Public Health 2008;55:431–5.
34. Murray KO, Holmes KC, Hanlon CA. Rabies in vaccinated dogs and cats in the United States, 1997-2001. J Amer Vet Med Assoc 2009;235:691–5.
35. Charleton KM, Webster WA, Casey GA. Skunk rabies. In: Baer GM, editor. The natural history of rabies. 2nd edition. Boca Raton (FL): CRC Press; 1991. p. 307–24.
36. Blanton JD, Palmer D, Rupprecht CE. Rabies surveillance in the United States during 2009. J Am Vet Med Assoc 2010;237:646–57.
37. National Association of State Public Health Veterinarians, Centers for Disease Control and Prevention. Compendium of animal rabies prevention and control, 2008: National Association of State Public Health Veterinarians, Inc. (NASPHV). MMWR Recomm Rep 2008;57:1–9.
38. McQuiston J, Yager PA, Smith JS, et al. Epidemiologic characteristics of rabies virus variants in dogs and cats in the United States, 1999. J Am Vet Med Assoc 2001;218:1939–42.
39. Clark KA, Neill SU, Smith JS, et al. Epizootic canine rabies transmitted by coyotes in south Texas. J Am Vet Med Assoc 1994;204:536–40.
40. Eng TR, Fishbein DB. Epidemiologic factors, clinical findings, and vaccination status of rabies in cats and dogs in the United States in 1988. National Study Group on Rabies. J Am Vet Med Assoc 1990;197:201–9.
41. Tizard I, Ni Y. Use of serologic testing to assess immune status of companion animals. J Am Vet Med Assoc 1998;213:54–60.
42. Greene CE, Rupprecht CE. Rabies and other lyssavirus infections. In: Greene CE, editor. Infectious diseases of the dog and cat. 3rd edition. Philadelphia: Saunders Elsevier; 2006. p. 167–83.
43. Rupprecht CE, Gilbert J, Pitts R, et al. Evaluation of an inactivated rabies virus vaccine in domestic ferrets. J Am Vet Med Assoc 1990;196:1614–6.
44. Bender JB, Shulman SA; Animals in Public Contact subcommittee; National Association of State Public Health Veterinarians. Reports of zoonotic disease outbreaks associated with animal exhibits and availability of recommendations for preventing zoonotic disease transmission from animals to people in such settings. J Am Vet Med Assoc 2004;224:1105–9.
45. Wilson PJ, Oertli EH, Hunt PR, et al. Evaluation of a postexposure rabies prophylaxis protocol for domestic animals in Texas: 2000-2009. J Am Vet Med Assoc 2010;237:1395–1401.
46. Johnson DH, Tinline RR. Rabies control in wildlife. In: Jackson AC, Wunner WH, editors. Rabies. San Diego (CA): Academic Press; 2002. p. 446–71.
47. MacInnes CD, Smith SM, Tinline RR, et al. Elimination of rabies from red foxes in eastern Ontario. J Wildl Dis 2001;37:119–32.
48. Rosatte RC, Power MJ, Donovan D, et al. Elimination of arctic variant rabies in red foxes, metropolitan Toronto. Emerg Infect Dis 2007;13:25–7.

49. Sidwa TJ, Wilson PJ, Moore GM, et al. Evaluation of oral rabies vaccination programs for control of rabies epizootics in coyotes and gray foxes: 1995–2003. J Am Vet Med Assoc. 2005;227:785–92.
50. Shwiff SA, Kirkpatrick KA, Sterner RT. Economic evaluation of a Texas oral rabies vaccination program for control of a domestic dog-coyote rabies epizootic: 1995–2006. J Am Vet Med Assoc 2008;233:1736–41.
51. Fearneyhough MG, Wilson PJ, Clark KA, et al. Results of an oral rabies vaccination program for coyotes. J Am Vet Med Assoc 1998;212:498–502.
52. Slate D, Rupprecht CE, Rooney JA, et al. Status of oral rabies vaccination in wild carnivores in the United States. Virus Res 2005;111:68–76.
53. Sterner RT, Meltzer MI, Shwiff SA, et al. Tactics and economics of wildlife oral rabies vaccination, Canada and the United States. Emerg Infect Dis 2009;15:1176–84.
54. Manning SE, Rupprecht CE, Fishbein D, et al; Advisory Committee on Immunization Practices Centers for Disease Control and Prevention (CDC). Human Rabies Prevention–United States, 2008: recommendations of the Advisory Committee on Immunization Practices. MMWR Recomm Rep 2008;57:1–28.
55. Morimoto K, Patel M, Corisdeo S, et al. Characterization of a unique variant of bat rabies virus responsible for newly emerging human cases in North America. Proc Natl Acad Sci U S A 1996;93:5653–8.
56. WHO Expert Consultation on Rabies. World Health Organ Tech Rep Ser 2005;931: 1–88.
57. Blanton JD, Robertson K, Palmer D, et al. Rabies surveillance in the United States during 2008. J Am Vet Med Assoc 2009;235:676–89.
58. Manning SE, Rupprecht CE, Fishbein D, et al; Advisory Committee on Immunization Practices Centers for Disease Control and Prevention (CDC). Human Rabies Prevention–United States, 2008: recommendations of the Advisory Committee on Immunization Practices. MMWR Recomm Rep 2008;57;1–28.
59. Griego RD, Rosen T, Orengo IF, et al. Dog, cat, and human bites: A review. J Am Acad Dermatol 1995;33:1019–29.
60. Fishbein DB, Sawyer LA, Reid-Sanden FL, et al. Administration of human diploid-cell rabies vaccine in the gluteal area. N Engl J Med 1988;318:124–5.
61. Rupprecht CE, Briggs D, Brown CM, et al; Centers for Disease Control and Prevention. Use of a reduced (4-dose) vaccine schedule for postexposure prophylaxis to prevent human rabies: recommendations of the advisory committee on immunization practices. MMWR Recomm Rep 2010;59:1–9.
62. Bryceson AD, Greenwood BM, Warrell DA, et al. Demonstration during life of rabies antigen in humans. J Infect Dis 1975;131:71–4.
63. Blenden DC, Creech W, Torres-Anjel MJ. Use of immunofluorescence examination to detect rabies virus in the skin of humans with clinical encephalitis. J Infect Dis 1986;154:698–701.
64. Crepin P, Audry L, Rotivel Y, et al. Intravital diagnosis of human rabies by PCR using saliva and cerebrospinal fluid. J Clin Microbiol 1998;36:1117–21.
65. Arai YT, Yamada K, Kameoka Y, et al. Nucleoprotein gene analysis of fixed and street rabies virus variants using RT-PCR. Arch Virol 1997;142:1787–96.
66. Nadin-Davis SA. Polymerase chain reaction protocols for rabies virus discrimination. J Virol Methods1998;75:1–8.
67. Smith JS, Yager PA, Baer GM. A rapid reproducible test for determining rabies neutralizing antibody. Bull World Health Organ 1973;48:535–41.
68. Alvarez L, Fajardo R, Lopez E, et al. Partial recovery from rabies in a nine-year-old boy. Pediatr Infect Dis J 1994;13:1154–5.

69. Willoughby RE Jr, Tieves KS, Hoffman GM, et al. Survival after treatment of rabies with induction of coma. N Engl J Med 2005;352:2508–14.
70. Hattwick MA, Weis TT, Stechschulte CJ, et al. Recovery from rabies. A case report. Ann Intern Med 1972;76:931–42.
71. Centers for Disease Control and Prevention. Presumptive abortive human rabies - Texas, 2009. MMWR Morb Mortal Wkly Rep 2010;59:185–90.

Zoonoses of Rabbits and Rodents

William Allen Hill, DVM, MPH, DACLAM[a,b],*, Julie Paige Brown, DVM[c]

KEYWORDS
- Rabbit • Rodent • Zoonoses
- Disease prevention

INTRODUCTION

The American Veterinary Medical Association estimated that 68.7 million (59.5%) US households owned pets in 2006.[1] Rabbits and rodents have increased in popularity as companion animals and are often purchased as first pets for children due to their low cost, relative size, and perceived ease of care. In 2006, 1.9 million households owned rabbits and 2.1 million households owned rodents including, but not limited to, hamsters, guinea pigs, and gerbils.[2] Activities such as hunting and camping also allow for human interactions with wild rabbits and rodents. In 2006, the US Fish and Wildlife Service estimated that 4.8 million Americans hunted small game including rabbits and squirrels.[3] In many environments, feral rabbits and rodents live in close proximity to humans, domesticated animals, and other wildlife.

Because of the popularity of rabbits and rodents as pets and the frequency of human interaction with feral species, zoonoses of rabbits and rodents are a public health concern. Below we discuss common zoonotic pathogens of rabbits and rodents.

Rabbit and Rodent Zoonoses

Yersina pestis

The gram-negative coccobacillus, *Yersina pestis*, is the causative agent of human plague. In the US, important rodent reservoirs include prairie dogs (*Cynomys* spp), ground squirrels (*Spermophilus* spp), antelope ground squirrels (*Ammospermophilus* spp), chipmunks (*Tamias* spp), woodrats (*Neotoma* spp), and mice (*Peromyscus* spp). Morbidity and mortality rates are substantial in rabbits and susceptible rodents and approach 100%.[4] In the United States, human cases of plague are confined to

[a] Office of Laboratory Animal Care, University of Tennessee, Knoxville, TN, USA
[b] Department of Comparative Medicine, The University of Tennessee Institute of Agriculture, Knoxville, TN, USA
[c] The University of Tennessee College of Veterinary Medicine, Knoxville, TN, USA
* Corresponding author. 2431 Joe Johnson Drive, 336 Ellington Plant Science, Knoxville, TN 37996.
E-mail address: wahill@utk.edu

Vet Clin Exot Anim 14 (2011) 519-531
doi:10.1016/j.cvex.2011.05.009
1094-9194/11/$ – see front matter © 2011 Elsevier Inc. All rights reserved.

western states and 5–15 cases are reported each year.[5–7] Although sciurid rodents are the primary plague reservoirs in the US, at least 3 human cases have been reported in association with skinning or handling wild rabbit carcasses.[6,7] Fleas are a vector for plague and more than 1500 flea species have been reported to be infected with *Y pestis*.[5] Human infections generally occur via bite of an infected flea but may also occur via cutaneous abrasions or mucous membrane contact with infected aerosols. Forms of the disease in humans include bubonic plague, septicemic plague, and pneumonic plague.[8] Measures to control zoonotic transmission of plague include rodent and flea control, particularly in endemic areas. Care should also be exercised when processing wild, small mammal carcasses. In particular, handlers should wear gloves, surgical masks, and eye protection, and disinfect equipment following use. When possible, individuals should avoid handling sick or dead animals.

Francisella tularensis

Tularemia, also called rabbit fever or deerfly fever, is a zoonosis caused by the pleomorphic, gram-negative coccobacillus *Francisella tularensis*. *F tularensis* is highly infectious, and as few as 10 to 50 organisms can cause human disease.[9,10] Ticks and other blood sucking arthropods serve as the most important biological vectors in the United States.[11] US human cases have also been linked to contact with cats, dogs, sheep and wild animals, predominantly rabbits.[12–15] A single case has been associated with a pet hamster bite.[16] Wild rabbits and rodents with tularemia appear lethargic in the terminal phase and are often preyed upon by other animals, continuing the disease transmission.[11] Tularemia is a notifiable disease in the US and cases have been recorded in all states but Hawaii.[17] In humans, tularemia presents as a flu-like illness followed by 1 of 6 clinical syndromes. Forms of human tularemia include: ulceroglandular, glandular, oropharyngeal, oculoglandular, pneumonic, and typhoidal.[11] The ulceroglandular form occurs most commonly in the US and is characterized by ulcer formation at the site of inoculation and regional lymphadenopathy. Veterinarians should consider tularemia as a differential diagnosis in febrile animals with or without lymphadenopathy in areas where the disease is endemic. Care should be exercised when handling wild game carcasses. In particular, handlers should wear gloves, disinfect equipment following use, and cook all meat thoroughly. When possible, individuals should also avoid handling sick or dead animals. Tick control and measures to eliminate exposure to ticks will also reduce tularemia exposure risk. Individuals should also be aware that pet hamsters might be a potential source of tularemia.

Rabbit Zoonoses

Enterohemorrhagic Escherichia coli

Enterohemorrhagic *E coli* (EHEC) are food and water-borne pathogens associated with diarrhea, hemorrhagic colitis, and hemolytic uremic syndrome in humans. EHEC O157 is the most common serotype isolated from humans in the USA. EHEC O157 has been isolated from all levels of the bovine gastrointestinal tract and ruminants, particularly cattle, are considered the primary reservoir hosts.[18] EHEC strains have been also been isolated from other domesticated animals and wildlife.[19–21] Enteropathogenic *E coli* O145:H⁻ and EHEC O153:H⁻ were associated with an outbreak of hemorrhagic diarrhea and sudden death in a group of Dutch belted rabbits.[22] Further work isolated EHEC from rabbit feces and identified the rabbit as a reservoir host.[23] The zoonotic potential of rabbits as sources for human EHEC infections requires further investigation. Human EHEC infections result from fecal-oral exposures including ingestion of contaminated food or water, direct contact with shedding animals, and direct contact with environmental contaminants. To reduce zoonotic transmission of EHEC, individuals should thoroughly wash their hands with soap and water after handling rabbits, their cages or other cage implements, and their bedding. Individuals should also avoid eating or drinking when handling rabbits.

Cryptosporidium spp

Cryptosporidium spp have been identified in over 150 mammalian hosts including rabbits.[24] Cryptosporidium spp cause mainly diarrheal diseases in infected humans and neonatal animals. Major pathogenic species include C hominus (humans) and C. parvum (humans and neonatal animals). In 2008, Cryptosporidium spp rabbit genotype was identified as the etiologic agent responsible for an outbreak of waterborne human cryptosporidiosis occurring in Northamptonshire, England.[25] A wild rabbit that gained access to the water treatment process was identified as the source of contamination. Rabbits infected with Cryptosporidium spp are usually asymptomatic.[26] The prevalence of Cryptosporidium spp in wild rabbits is estimated at up to 5%, although additional epidemiological studies are needed.[24] Rabbits are likely susceptible to infection with Cryptosporidium rabbit genotype, C parvum, and C meleagridis all of which are human pathogens.[24] The role of rabbits as a potential source of zoonotic cryptosporidiosis should be considered. Practices to reduce zoonotic transmission of Cryptosporidium spp include thorough hand washing and preventing animal fecal contamination of water supplies.

Encephalitozoon cuniculi

Encephalitozoon cuniculi is an obligate, intracellular, spore-forming, microsporidial parasite that has been documented in rabbits, rodents, carnivores, primates, and birds.[27,28] The agent was formerly named Nosema cuniculi. In rabbits, encephalitozoonosis is usually latent, yet clinical signs may include convulsions, tremors, torticollis, paresis, and coma. Lesions including pitting of renal cortices, granulomatous inflammation of the kidney, lung, liver, brain, and spinal cord, and cataract formation have all been reported in rabbits with E cuniculi infection.[26,29] Routes of transmission are unknown; however, the organism has been found in the urine of infected rabbits. E cuniculi is a zoonotic parasite, and infections have been reported in immunosuppressed AIDS patients.[30] Encephalitozoonosis should be suspected in severely immunocompromised patients presenting with multi-organ involvement, including renal failure, keratoconjunctivitis, fever, and respiratory and neurologic symptoms. Control of E cuniculi in a rabbitry should involve identification and elimination of infected animals and environmental disinfection. Lysol, Formalin, ethanol, and sodium hypoclorite have shown microbicidal activity against Encephalitozoon.[29]

Pasteurella spp

Pasteurella spp are gram-negative, non–spore-forming coccobacilli and are found as part of the normal flora of the upper respiratory tract of some mammals. Pasteurella multocida is the causative agent of pasteurellosis, a common disease of rabbits. Clinical signs of Pasteurella multocida infection in rabbits include: rhinitis, sinusitis, pneumonia, otis media, otitis interna, conjunctivitis, abscess formation, genital infection, and septicemia.[29] Infected rabbits may also be asymptomatic. In humans, clinical signs associated with Pasteurella infection include necrotizing fasciitis, septic arthritis, osteomyelitis, and less frequently, sepsis, shock, and meningitis.[31] Individuals at increased risk for Pasteurella spp infection include infants, pregnant women, and immunocompromised patients. Most human Pasteurella spp infections are caused by dog or cat bites. There is a single report describing human *Pasteurella multocida* infection following a rabbit bite.[32] Local cleansing and antisepsis of animal bite wounds is recommended to prevent zoonotic transmission of *Pasteurella multocida*. Antibiotic therapy may be warranted in some cases.

Coxiella burnetti

Q fever is caused by the bacterium *Coxiella burnetii*, a small, gram-negative, pleomorphic rod. The reservoirs of *C burnetii* are only partially known and include mammals, birds, and arthropods, mainly ticks.[33] *C burnetii* multiplies in the gut cells of ticks and is shed in tick feces; however, most human infections do not result from tick exposure. *C burnettii* is shed in the urine, feces, milk, and placental tissues of domestic ungulates. The most commonly identified sources of human infection are infected cattle, sheep, and goats.[33] Human cases have also been associated with pregnant cats, pigeon feces, and wild rabbits.[34–36] Q fever pneumonia was reported in 4 patients with a history of exposure to wild rabbits.[36] Routes of human transmission include aerosolization, ingestion, and less commonly person to person transmission. In humans, Q fever often presents as a flu-like illness with fever and headache and a nonproductive cough with pneumonia. Hepatitis, nephritis, epicarditis, and endocarditis may also occur.[33] Effective tick control strategies and good hygiene practices can decrease *C burnettii* environmental contamination. Zoonotic risk can further be reduced by appropriate handling of fetal tissues and contaminated bedding and exercising caution when processing wild rabbit carcasses.

Cheyletiella spp

Cheyletiella spp are nonburrowing mites of rabbits, cats, dogs, and humans.[37] *Cheyletiella* spp live in the keratin layer of the epidermis and feed on surface debris and tissue fluids.[38] *Cheyletiella* spp reported to occur on rabbits include *C parasitovorax*, *C takahasii*, *C ochotonae*, and *C johnsoni*.[29] In rabbits, *Cheyletiella* spp infections occur most commonly on the dorsal trunk and scapular areas and may be asymptomatic or cause a mild alopecia and seborrhea sicca over the infected area.[26,29] Mites can be identified by microscopic examination of superficial skin scrapings. Topical acaricides and parenteral ivermectin are effective treatments to control infestations in rabbits. Transmission to humans is likely via direct contact. When in close physical contact with humans, *Cheyletiella* spp "bite and run", and then rapidly return to their non-human animal host.[38] The primary lesion of human *Cheyletiella* infestation is reported as a small, pruritic, erythematous papule surmounted by a fragile vesicle and is most commonly found on the forearms, breast, and abdomen.[37,38] Disease in humans is typically self-limiting. Veterinary examination of pets is advisable if companion animal owners have unexplained papular dermatitis.

Dermatophytosis

In rabbits, the fungus most commonly identified with clinical dermatophytosis is *Trichophyton mentagrophytes*; however, *Microsporum canis* has also been reported to occur in rabbits.[39] Dermatophyte lesions are generally located around the head and ears with secondary spread to the feet and are characterized by patchy alopecia with crusting. Lesions are typically circular, erythematous, and pruritic. Consistent with dermatophytosis in other species, the lesion expands radially with central healing. Griseofluvin and copper sulfate have been reported as treatment for rabbit dermatophytosis.[29] The disease is easily transmitted to susceptible humans and rabbits with suspected dermatophyte infections should be isolated due to potential risks to humans and other animals. *T. mentagrophytes* spores can be isolated from infected rabbits, including asymptomatic carriers, rabbit nests, and the surrounding environment and all may be important sources of zoonoses transmission. *T mentagrophytes* of rabbit origin has been reported to cause a family incidence of kerion in humans.[40]

Rodent Zoonoses

Bartonella spp

Bartonella spp are gram-negative bacteria which are mainly transmitted by vectors and cause a long-lasting intra-erythrocytic bacteremia. Among the 13 *Bartonella* species or subspecies known or suspected to be pathogenic for humans, four have been isolated from cats.[41] Cat scratch disease is the most common zoonoses caused by *Bartonella* spp An increasing number of animal reservoir hosts, including rodents, have been identified for various *Bartonella* spp.[42] *Bartonella* spp were isolated from the blood of 42.2% (119/279) of wild rodents tested in the southeastern United States.[43] Additionally, exotic small mammals used in the pet trade may be reservoirs of zoonotic *Bartonella* spp.[44] Of the rodent-associated *Bartonella* spp, *B elizabethae*, *B grahamii*, *B visonii* subsp *arupensis*, and *B washoensis* have been implicated in human infections of endocarditis, neuroretinitis, pyrexia and endocarditis, and myocarditis, respectively.[44] The mechanisms by which humans acquire *Bartonella* infections from rodents are unknown. Likely modes of transmission would include direct contact with bacteria shed from rodents and vector transmission by rodent ectoparasites.[45]

Leptospira spp

Leptospirosis, a worldwide public health problem, is an acute bacterial infection caused by pathogenic spirochetes of the genus *Leptospira*. Over 250 *Leptospira* serovars are known and each serovar has a preferred animal host.[46] The most common *Leptospira* in rats is *L icterohemorrhagiae*.[47] Leptospires are excreted into the environment through the urine of infected animals; human infections are generally acquired through direct or environmental contact with infected urine. Humans are susceptible to a large number of *Leptospira* serovars including *L icterohemorrhagiae*. A single report describes a case of human *L icterohemorrhagiae* infection acquired from pet rats.[46] Wild rodents are often identified as the source of human infection. In humans, the majority of leptospiral infections are subclinical or mild; however, a small proportion of patients develop severe icteric illness with renal failure or hemorrhagic pneumonitis.[48] *Leptospira* infections in rats are subclinical and animals present with minimal or no lesions.[47] To reduce the risk of acquiring leptospirosis, individuals should avoid drinking or swimming in water potentially contaminated with animal urine. Individuals with occupational or recreational exposure to contaminated water or soil should wear protective clothing including gloves, masks, and footwear.[49] Additionally, individuals should thoroughly wash their hands with soap and water after handling pet rodents, their cages or other cage implements, and their bedding.

Salmonella spp

Salmonella spp are gram-negative bacteria that cause gastroenteritis, bactermia, and subsequent focal infection. *Salmontella* Typhimurium is the serotype most commonly associated with animal and human disease.[5] More than 95% of cases of *Salmonella* infection are foodborne and salmonellosis accounts for approximately 30% of US foodborne illness associated deaths.[50] Many human *Salmonella* infections are acquired by contact with animals. A multistate human outbreak of multidrug-resistant *Salmonella* enteric serotype Typhimurium infections was associated with exposure to pet hamsters, mice, and rats.[51] A second multi-state human outbreak of *S.* Typhimurium was associated with feeding frozen vacuum packed rodents to pet snakes.[52] The snakes acquired *S* Typhimurium from frozen feed mice and human transmission likely occurred through contact with the snakes, their feed, or contaminated environmental surfaces. Clinical illness associated with *Salmonella* infections in mice and rats is rare but may include diarrhea, anorexia, weight loss, conjunctivitis, and variable mortality.[47,53] In hamsters, salmonellosis can cause severe disease with morbidity and mortality.[54] Owners should be aware that rodents can shed salmonella and should expect rodent feces to be potentially infectious. Additionally, individuals feeding rodents to reptiles should also be aware that feeder animals can be infectious and can transmit *Salmonella* infections to reptiles. To reduce zoonotic transmission of *Salmonella*, individuals should thoroughly wash their hands with soap and water after handling rodents and rodent-fed reptiles, their cages or other cage implements, and their bedding.

Streptobacillus moniliformis

The gram-negative, pleomorphic rod, *Streptobacillus moniliformis*, is the primary cause of US human rat bite fever (RBF) cases. *Spirillum minus* causes RBF in Africa and Asia.[55] *S moniliformis* inhabits the nasopharynx, middle ear, and respiratory tract of wild rats (*Rattus norvegicus*) and is also present in the blood and urine of infected animals. *S moniliformis* does not cause clinical signs in rats.[56] *S moniliformis* may be transmitted to humans from a bite or scratch from an infected rat, handling of an infected rat, or ingestion of food or water contaminated with infected rat excreta.[57] Mice and gerbils may also be reservoirs of *S moniliformis*. Initial symptoms of *S moniliformis* infection in humans are non-specific and include fever, chills, myalgia, headache, and vomiting and typically occur within 7 days of exposure. Patients may also develop a maculopapular rash on the extremities or septic arthritis followed by arthralgia.[58] RBF carries a mortality rate of 7–10% among untreated patients.[57] Individuals at risk for RBF include those with recreational or occupational exposure to rats and children living in rat infested urban dwellings or rural areas. To reduce exposure to *S moniliformis*, individuals should wear gloves, practice regular hand washing, and avoid hand-to-mouth contact when handling rats or cleaning rat enclosures. If bitten by a rat, individuals should promptly clean and disinfect the wound, seek medical attention, and report their exposure history.[57]

Rickettsia akari

Rickettsia akari, a member of the spotted fever group *Rickettsia*, is the cause of the mite-borne zoonosis, rickettsialpox. Rickettsialpox was first identified in New York City in 1946 and most US recognized cases continue to originate from this area.[59,60] Rickettsialpox is most likely to occur in crowded urban areas with mouse infested housing.[61] The house mouse (*Mus musculus*) is the natural host *R akari* and the house mouse mite (*Liponysoides sanguineus*) has been identified as the primary vector. Humans are incidental hosts of *L sanguineus* and become infected when bitten by mites infected with *R akari*. Other mite and rodent species may also be involved in the cycle.[62] In humans, rickettsialpox is characterized by an ulcerated primary lesion or eschar at the site of inoculation, followed by a systemic illness that includes fever, headache, and a generalized papulovesicular rash.[60] Rickettsialpox should be considered in any patient with fever and a papulovesicular eruption.

Rickettsia typhi

Rickettsia typi, an obligate intracellular gram-negative organism, is the causative agent of murine or endemic typhus. Rats (*Rattus rattus* and *Rattus norvegicus)* are the primary reservoirs of *R typi*; however, other mammals including house mice (Mus musculus), opossums, skunks, cats, and dogs can maintain infection.[63] Vectors include the rat flea, *Xenopsylla cheopis*, and the cat flea, *Ctenocephalides felis*.[64] Humans acquire infection mainly when an infected flea bites and feces are inoculated into the bite site.[65] Currently less than 100 cases are reported annually in the US and most cases are limited to Texas and Southern California.[66] Clinical signs of human *R typhi* infection include fever, headache, and myalgias, followed by a discrete maculopulular rash. The mortality rate for murine typhus is low (1%) with appropriate antibiotics.[67] Prevention of murine typhus includes use of flea preventive on dogs and cats, exterminating household rodents, eliminating rodent habitats in or near homes, using pesticides to limit flea infestations, and avoiding wild animals including feral cats and opossums, and using insect repellents.[63]

Hantaviruses

Hantaviruses are rodent viruses that have been identified as etiologic agents of 2 human diseases: hemorrhagic fever with renal syndrome and hantavirus pulmonary syndrome. Hemorrhagic fever with renal syndrome occurs outside the Americas. In 1993, hantavirus pulmonary syndrome (HPS), was identified among residents of the southwestern United States and has been subsequently recognized through the contiguous United States and the Americas.[68] HPS is a notifiable disease and as of December 2009, 537 cases of HPS had been reported to CDC, with a case-fatality rate of 36%.[69] Sin Nombre virus has been the cause of most HPS cases in North America. In the US, serological survey have identified hantavirus infections in the following species: rats (*Rattus norvegicus*), deer mice (*Peromyscus maniculatus*), white footed mice (*P leucopus*), meadow voles (*Microtus pennsylvanicus*), chipmunks (*Tamias* spp), cotton rats (*Sigmodon hispidus*), western harvest mice (*Reithrodontomys megalotis*), marsh rice rats (*Oryzomys palustris*), and pack rats (*Neotoma* spp).[5] Hantaviruses do not cause overt illness in their rodent hosts; however, infected rodents shed virus in saliva, urine, and feces for many weeks, months, or for life.[68] Transmission of hantaviruses to humans does not require direct contact with rodents. Human hantavirus infections are acquired by the respiratory route, most commonly through inhalation of virus-containing aerosols of rodent feces, saliva, or urine.[70] In humans, HPS typically has a 2–10 day prodrome with nonspecific viral symptoms and patients proceed rapidly to respiratory failure due to capillary leakage into the lungs, followed by shock and cardiac complications.[5] Recommendations to reduce zoonotic risk for hantavirus infection include trapping and excluding rodents and using personal protective equipment such as masks and eye protection when handling potentially infected rodents or disturbing areas of rodent infestation.[69]

Lymphocytic choriomeningitis virus

Lymphocytic choriomeningitis virus (LCMV) is a RNA virus and belongs to the genus *Arenavirus*. Wild mice are the natural reservoir of LCMV, but LCVM is also known to infect hamsters and guinea pigs.[71] In mice, clinical signs of natural LCMV are minimal but may include runting in neonates, reduced litter size, and wasting in adult mice.[53] In humans, LCMV infection is usually asymptomatic or mild and self limiting; however, acute meningoencephalities and congenital malformation of the CNS and eye may occur.[72] Immunocompromised individuals and women in the first or second trimester of pregnancy are at increased risk of developing severe complications following infection.[54] Most human cases of LCMV are associated with the wild house mouse.[71,73] Humans usually become infected with LCMV through direct contact with infected rodents, including bites, or through inhalation of infectious rodent excreta

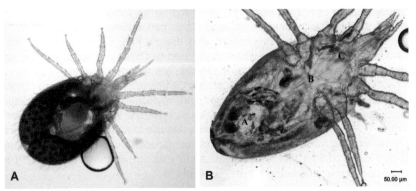

Fig. 1. The tropical rat mite, *Ornithonyssus bacoti*. (*A*) Dorsal view of a blood engorged mite. (*B*) Ventral view of mite with anal (A), genital (B), and sternal (C) shields labeled.

and secreta.[74] In 2005, a cluster of 4 human cases of LCMV and three fatalities among organ transplant recipients were attributed to a LCMV infected donor. The organ donor was determined to have had contact with a pet hamster infected with an LCMV stain identical to the strain detected in the organ recipients.[75] Zoonotic risk of LCMV infection can be reduced by hand washing after handling pet rodents or cleaning their cages. Pet rodents should never be permitted contact with wild rodents, their droppings, or their nests. Pregnant women and immunocompromised individuals may wish to avoid contact with rodents, especially wild rodents.[76]

Monkeypox virus
Monkeypox virus is an orthopoxvirus and causes human monkeypox, a rare viral zoonosis endemic to central and western Africa. In 2003, an outbreak of human monkey pox in the US was identified and attributed to exposure to infected captive prairie dogs.[77] Monkeypox virus was likely introduced to the US through an import shipment of Gambian giant rats and other exotic African rodents, which were comingled with other mammals, including prairie dogs, in an Illinois pet distribution center.[77,78] Most human cases had direct physical contact with infected animals and infection likely resulted from bites, scratches, or open wounds.[79] Clinical signs of monkeypox in the infected prairie dogs included, anorexia, wasting, respiratory signs, blephritis, ocular discharge, papular skin lesions and sudden death.[78,80] Monkeypox in humans generally presents as fever and malaise followed by rash and lymphadenopathy.[81] Health-care providers and public health practitioners who suspect monkeypox in animals or humans should report such cases to their state and local health departments.

Ornithonyssus bacoti
The tropical rat mite, *Ornithonyssus bacoti*, is an obligate blood-feeding parasite with world-wide distribution (**Fig. 1**). Natural host of *O bacoti* include several species of rats and mice, hamsters, gerbils, voles, and other wild rodents. Nonrodent hosts include cats and other wild and domestic carnivores, some birds, opossums, and humans.[82] In laboratory mice, severe *O bactoi* infestations have been association with decreased litter production, anemia, and death.[83,84] Two recent Ornithonyssus bacoti outbreaks have been described in laboratory mice.[82,85] In most instances, outbreaks of *O. bacoti* are recognized only when humans are attacked in the absence of an

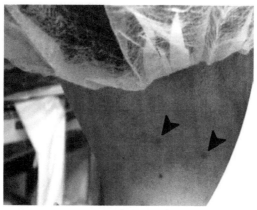

Fig. 2. Papular lesions *(arrowheads)* on the neck of the research technician.

animal host.[86] The non-specific dermatitis caused by the mite's attack is commonly referred to as "rat-mite dermatitis" and results from an inflammatory reaction to the mite's saliva as it takes a blood meal (**Fig. 2**). Pet hamsters have been associated with human cases of rat mite dermatitis.[87] *O bacoti* can also harbor pathogens including *R typhi, R acari, C burnetti, F tularensis,* Eastern equine encephalitis virus, hemorrhagic fever with renal syndrome virus, *Borrelia burgdorferi,* and *Y pestis,* raising additional public health concerns.[88] Permethrin impregnanted cotton balls have been shown to eliminate *O bacoti* from laboratory mice.[82,85] Rodent owners and individuals with occupational exposure to rodents with unexplained dermatitis should consult a physician.

SUMMARY

The article highlights the significant role of rabbits and rodents in the transmission of a large number of zoonotic diseases. Although most of the aforementioned zoonoses are rare, veterinarians, physicians, and public health practitioners should be knowledgeable of the clinical presentation of these diseases and practices to reduce individual risk. Education of rodent and rabbit owners and individuals with occupational or recreational exposures to these species is paramount to reduce the prevalence of zoonoses associated with rabbit and rodent exposure.

REFERENCES

1. American Veterinary Medical Association. Total pet ownership and pet population: all pets. In: US pet ownership and demographics sourcebook. Schaumburg: American Veterinary Medical Association; 2007. p. 7–12.
2. American Veterinary Medical Association. Total pet ownership and pet population: specialty and exotic pet ownership. In: US pet ownership and demographics sourcebook. Schaumburg: American Veterinary Medical Association; 2007. p. 45–7.
3. United States Fish and Wildlife Service Web site. Hunting statistics and economics. Available at: http://www.fws.gov/hunting/huntstat.html. Accessed May 12, 2011.
4. Orloski KA, Lathrop SL. Plague: a veterinary perspective. J Am Vet Med Assoc 2003;222:444–8.
5. Fox JG, Newcomer CE, Rozmiarek H. Selected Zoonoses. In: Fox JG, Anderson LC, Loew FM, et al, editors. Laboratory animal medicine. 2nd edition. New York: Academic Press; 2002. p. 1059–105.

6. Centers for Disease Control and Prevention (CDC). Human plague–four states, 2006. MMWR Morb Mortal Wkly Rep 2006;55:940–3.

7. Centers for Disease Control. Human plague–United States, 1988. MMWR Morb Mortal Wkly Rep 1988;37:653–6.

8. Prentice MB, Rahalison L. Plague. Lancet 2007;369:1196–207.

9. Saslaw S, Eigelsbach HT, Wilson HE, et al. Tularemia vaccine study. I. Intracutaneous challenge. Arch Intern Med 1961;107:689–701.

10. Saslaw S, Eigelsbach HT, Prior JA, et al. Tularemia vaccine study. II. Respiratory challenge. Arch Intern Med 1961;107:702–14.

11. Feldman KA. Tularemia. J Am Vet Med Assoc 2003;222: 725–30.

12. Centers for Disease Control. Tularemia associated with domestic cats–Georgia, New Mexico. MMWR Morb Mortal Wkly Rep 1982;31:39–41.

13. Rumble CT. Pneumonic tularemia following the shearing of a dog. J Med Assoc Ga 1972;61:355.

14. Senol M, Ozcan A, Karincaoglu Y, et al. Tularemia: a case transmitted from sheep. Cutis 1999;63:49–51.

15. Ryan-Poirier K, Whitehead PY, Leggiadro RJ. An unlucky rabbit's foot. Pediatrics 1990;85:598–600.

16. Centers for Disease Control and Prevention. Tularemia associated with a hamster bite–Colorado, 2004. MMWR Morb Mortal Wkly Rep 2005;53:1202–3.

17. Centers for Disease Control and Prevention. Tularemia–United States, 1990–2000. MMWR Morb Mortal Wkly Rep 2002;51:181–4.

18. Garcia A, Fox JG, Besser TE. Zoonotic enterohemorrhagic Escherichia coli: A One Health perspective. ILAR 2010;51:221–32.

19. Hancock DD, Besser TE, Rice DH, et al. Multiple sources of Escherichia coli O157 in feedlots and dairy farms in the northwestern USA. Prev Med 1998;35:11–9.

20. Cornick NA, Vukhac H. Indirect transmission of Escherichia coli O157:H7 occurs readily among swine but not among sheep. Appl Environ Microbiol 2008;74: 2488–91.

21. Chapman PA, Siddons CA, Gerdan Malo AT, et al. A 1-year study of Escherichia coli O157 in cattle, sheep, pigs and poultry. Epidemiol Infect 1997;119:245–50.

22. García A, Marini RP, Feng Y, et al. A naturally occurring rabbit model of enterohemorrhagic Escherichia coli-induced disease. J Infect Dis 2002;186:1683–6.

23. Garcia A, Fox JG. The rabbit as a new reservoir host of enterohemorrhagic Escherichia coli. Emerg Infect Dis 2003;9:1592–6.

24. Robinson G, Chalmers RM. The European rabbit (Oryctolagus cuniculus), a source of zoonotic cryptosporidiosis. Zoonoses Public Health 2010;57:e1–13.

25. Health Protection Report. Outbreak of cryptosporidiosis associated with a water contamination incident in the East Midlands. Vol. 2, No. 29. Available at http://www.hpa.org.uk/hpr/archives/2008/news2908.htm. Accessed May 12, 2011.

26. Percy DH, Barthold SW. Rabbit. In: Pathology of laboratory rodents and rabbits. 3rd edition. Ames: Blackwell Publishing Professional; 2007. p. 253–307.

27. Deplazes P, Mathis A, Baumgartner R, et al. Immunologic and molecular characteristics of Encephalitozoon-like microsporidia isolated from humans and rabbits indicate that Encephalitozoon cuniculi is a zoonotic parasite. Clin Infect Dis 1996;22: 557–9.

28. Dipineto L, Rinaldi L, Santaniello A, et al. Serological survey for antibodies to Encephalitozoon cuniculi in pet rabbits in Italy. Zoonoses Public Health 2008;173–5.

29. Suckow MA, Brammer DW, Rush HG, et al. Biology and diseases of rabbits. In: Fox JG, Anderson LC, Loew FM, et al, editors. Laboratory animal medicine. 2nd edition. New York: Academic Press; 2002. p. 328–63.

30. Fournier S, Liguory O, Sarfati C. Disseminated infection due to Encephalitozoon cuniculi in a patient with AIDS: case report and review. HIV Med 2000;1:155–61.
31. Oehler RL, Velez AP, Mizrachi M, et al. Bite-related and septic syndromes caused by cats and dogs. Lancet 2009;9:439–47.
32. Boisvert PL, Fousek MD. Human infection with Pasteurella lepiseptica following a rabbit bite. JAMA 1941;116:1902–3.
33. Angelakis E, Raoult D. Q Fever. Vet Microbiol 2010;140:297–309.
34. Marrie TJ, Raoult D. Update on Q fever, including Q fever endocarditis. Curr Clin Top Infect Dis 2002;22:97–124.
35. Stein A, Raoult D. Pigeon pneumonia in Provence: a bird borne Q fever outbreak. Clin Infect Dis 1999;29:617–20.
36. Marrie TJ, Schlech WF 3rd, Williams JC, et al. Q fever pneumonia associated with exposure to wild rabbits. Lancet 1986;1:427–9.
37. Cohen SR. Cheyletiella dermatitis. A mite infestation of rabbit, cat, dog, and man. Arch Dermatol 1980;116:435–7.
38. Wagner R, Stallmeister N. Cheyletiella dermatitis in humans, dogs and cats. B J Dermatol 2000;143:1110–2.
39. Cafarchia C, Camarda A, Coccioli C, et al. Epidemiology and risk factors for dermatophytoses in rabbit farms. Med Mycol 2010;48:975–80.
40. Van Rooij P, Detandt M, Nolard N. Trichophyton mentagrophytes of rabbit origin causing family incidence of kerion: an environmental study. Mycoses 2006;49: 426–30.
41. Chomel BB, Kasten RW. Bartonellosis, an increasingly recognized zoonosis. J Appl Microbiol 2010;109:743–50.
42. Breitschwerdt EB, Maggi RG, Chomel BB, et al. Bartonellosis: an emerging infectious disease of zoonotic importance to animals and human beings. J Vet Emerg Crit Care 2010;20:8–30.
43. Kosoy MY, Regnery RL, Tzianabos T, et al. Distribution, diversity, and host specificity of Bartonella in rodents from the Southeastern United States. Am J Trop Med Hyg 1997;57:578–8.
44. Inoue K, Maruyama S, Kabeya H, et al. Exotic small mammals as potential reservoirs of zoonotic Bartonella spp. Emerg Infect Dis 2009;15:526–32.
45. Comer JA, Diaz T, Vlahov D, et al. Evidence of rodent-associated Bartonella and Rickettsia infections among intravenous drug users from central and east Harlem, New York City. Am J Trop Med Hyg 2001;65: 855–60.
46. Gaudie CM, Featherstone CA, Phillips WS, et al. Human Leptospira interrogans serogroup icterohaemorrhagiae infection (Weil's disease) acquired from pet rats. Vet Rec 2008;163:599–601.
47. Percy DH, Barthold SW. Rat. In: Pathology of laboratory rodents and rabbits. 3rd edition. Ames (IA): Blackwell Publishing Professional: 2007. p. 125–78.
48. Vijayachari P, Sugunan AP, Shriram AN. Leptospirosis: an emerging global public health problem. J Biosci 2008;33:557–69.
49. Centers for Disease Control and Prevention Web site. Leptospirosis. Available at: http://www.cdc.gov/ncidod/dbmd/diseaseinfo/leptospirosis_g.htm#Can leptospirosis be prevented. Accessed January 1, 2011.
50. Mead PS, Slutsker L, Dietz V, et al. Food-related illness and death in the United States. Emerg Infect Dis 1999;5:607–25.
51. Swanson SJ, Snider C, Braden CR, et al. Multidrug-resistant Salmonella enterica serotype Tymphimurium associated with pet rodents. New Engl J Med 2007;356: 21–8.

52. Fuller CC, Jawahir SL, Leano FT, et al. A multi-state Salmonella Typhimurium outbreak associated with frozen vacuum-packed rodents used to feed snakes. Zoonoses Public Health 2008;55;481–7.

53. Percy DH, Barthold SW. Mouse. In: Pathology of laboratory rodents and rabbits. 3rd edition. Ames (IA): Blackwell Publishing Professional: 2007. p. 3–124.

54. Percy DH, Barthold SW. Hamster. In: Pathology of laboratory rodents and rabbits. 3rd edition. Ames (IA): Blackwell Publishing Professional: 2007. p. 179–205.

55. Centers for Disease Control and Prevention Web site. Rat-bite fever: technical information. Available at: http://www.cdc.gov/nczved/divisions/dfbmd/diseases/ratbite_fever/technical.html. Accessed May 12, 2011.

56. Kohn DF, Clifford CB. Biology and diseases of rats. In: Fox JG, Anderson LC, Loew FM, et al, editors. Laboratory animal medicine. 2nd edition. New York: Academic Press; 2002. p. 121–65.

57. Centers for Disease Control and Prevention. Fatal rat-bite fever–Florida and Washington 2003. MMWR Morb Mortal Wkly Rep 2005;53:1198–202.

58. Freels LK, Elliott SP. Rat bite fever: three case reports and a literature review. Clin Pediatr 2004;43:291–5.

59. Huebner RJ, Stamps P, Armstrong C. Rickettsialpox—a newly recognized rickettsial disease. Public Health Rep 1946;62:1605–14.

60. Paddock CD, Koss T, Eremeeva MA, et al. Isolation of Rickettsia akari from eschars of patients with rickettsialpox. Am J Trop Med Hyg 2006;75:732–8.

61. Kass EM, Szaniawski WK, Levy H, et al. Rickettsialpox in a New York city hospital, 1980 to 1989. New Engl J Med 1994;331:1612–7.

62. Bennett SG, Comer JA, Smith HM, et al. Serologic evidence of a Rickettsia akari-like infection among wild-caught rodents in Orange County and humans in Los Angeles County, California. J Vector Ecol 2007;32:198–201.

63. Centers for Disease Control and Prevention. Outbreak of Rickettsia typhi infection - Austin, Texas, 2008. MMWR Morb Mortal Wkly Rep 2009;58:1267–70.

64. Fergie JE, Purcell K, Wanat D. Murine typhus in South Texas children. Pediatr Infect Dis J 2000;19:535–8.

65. Azad AF. Epidemiology of murine typhus. Ann Rev Entomol 1990;35:553–69.

66. Green JS, Singh J, Cheung M, et al. A cluster of pediatric endemic typhus cases in Orange County California. Pediatr Infect Dis J 2011;30:163–5.

67. Civen R, Ngo V. Murine typhus: an unrecognized suburban vectorbone disease. Clin Infect Dis 2008;46:913–8.

68. Mills JN, Corneli A, Young JC, et al. Hantavirus pulmonary syndrome–United States: updated recommendations for risk reduction. MMWR Recomm Rep 2002;51:1–12.

69. Centers for Disease Control and Prevention. Hantavirus pulmonary syndrome in five pediatric patients - four states, 2009. MMWR MMWR Morb Mortal Wkly Rep 2009;58:1409–12.

70. Lednicky JA. Hantaviruses, a short review. Arch Pathol Lab Med 2003;127:30–5.

71. Centers for Disease Control and Prevention. Update: interim guidance for minimizing risk for human lymphocytic choriomeningitis virus infection associated with pet rodents. MMWR Morb Mortal Wkly Rep 2005;54:799–801.

72. Emonet S, Retornaz K, Gonzalez JP, et al. Mouse-to-human transmission of variant lymphocytic choriomeningitis virus. Emerg Infect Dis 2007;13:472–5.

73. Jay MT, Glaser C, Fulhorst CF. The arenaviruses. J Am Vet Med Assoc 2005;227:904–15.

74. Charrel RN, de Lamballerie X. Zoonotic aspects of arenavirus infections. Vet Microbiol 2010;140:213–20.

75. Fischer SA, Graham MB, Kuehnert MJ, et al. Transmission of lymphocytic choriomeningitis virus by organ transplantation. N Engl J Med 2006;354:2235–49.
76. Hoey J. Lymphocytic choriomeningitis virus. CMAJ 2005;173:1033.
77. Centers for Disease Control and Prevention. Multistate outbreak of monkeypox–Illinois, Indiana, and Wisconsin, 2003. MMWR Morb Mortal Wkly Rep 2003;52: 537–40.
78. Reed KD, Melski JW, Graham MB, et al. The detection of monkeypox in humans in the western hemisphere. N Engl J Med 2004;350:342.
79. Bernard SM, Anderson SA. Qualitative assessment of risk for monkeypox associated with domestic trade in certain animal species, United States. Emerg Infect Dis 2006;12:1827–33.
80. Guarner J, Johnson BJ, Paddock CD, et al. Monkeypox transmission and pathogenesis in prairie dogs. Emerg Infect Dis 2004;10:426–31.
81. Di Giulio DB, Eckburg PB. Human monkeypox: an emerging zoonosis. Lancet 2004;4:15–25.
82. Hill WA, Randolph MM, Boyd KL, et al. Use of permethrin eradicated the tropical rat mite (Ornithonyssus bacoti) from a colony of mutagenized and transgenic mice. JAALAS 2005;44:31–4.
83. Keefe TJ, Scanlon JE, Wetherald LD. Ornithonyssus bacoti (Hirst) infestation in mouse and hamster colonies. Lab Anim Care 1964;14:366–9.
84. Harris JM, Stockton JJ. Eradication of the tropical rat mite Ornithonyssus bacoti (Hirst, 1913) from a colony of mice. Am J Vet Res 1960;21:316–8.
85. Cole JS, Sabol-Jones M, Karolewski B, et al. Ornithonyssus bacoti infestation and elimination from a mouse colony. Contemp Top Lab Anim Sci 2005;44:27–30.
86. Fishman HC. Rat mite dermatitis. Cutis 1988;42:414–6.
87. Creel NB, Crowe MA, Mullen GR. Pet hamsters as a source of rat mite dermatitis. Cutis 2003;71:457–61.
88. Baker DG. Parasites of rats and mice. In: Baker DG, editor. Flynn's parasites of laboratory animals. 2nd edition. Ames (IA): Blackwell Publishing; 2007. p. 303–97.

Zoonoses of Ferrets, Hedgehogs, and Sugar Gliders

Charly Pignon, DVM[a],*,
Jörg Mayer, Drmedvet, MSc, Dip ABVP (Exotic Companion Mammals)[b]

KEYWORDS

- Zoonoses • Ferrets • Hedgehogs • Sugar gliders

With urbanization, people live in close proximity to their pets. People often share living quarters and furniture with their pet companions, and this proximity carries a new potential for pathogen transmission. In addition to the change in lifestyle with our pets, new "exotic" pets are being introduced to the pet industry regularly. Often, we are unfamiliar with specific clinical signs of diseases in these new exotic pets or the routes of transmission of pathogens for the particular species.

Zoonoses are particularly important in the routine work of veterinarians. As veterinary practitioners, it is our duty to recognize and inform owners about the potential risk of a contracting a zoonotic disease from their pet. This article provides a review of zoonoses that occur naturally in ferrets, hedgehogs, and sugar gliders, including the occurrence and clinical symptoms of these diseases in humans.

BACTERIAL ZOONOSES

Salmonellosis

The genus *Salmonella* belongs to the family *Enterobacteriaceae*. It is made up of gram-negative, motile, facultatively anaerobic bacteria. *Salmonellae* grow between 46°F (8°C) and 113°F (45°C) and at a pH of 4 to 8. They do not survive at temperatures higher than 158°F (>70°C). These bacteria can resist dehydration for a very long time, both in feces and in foods for human and animal consumption. In addition, they can survive for several months in brine with 20% salinity. Except for serotypes *S* Typhi, *S* Paratyphi A, and *S* Paratyphi C, which are strictly human pathogens and whose only reservoir is man, all serotypes can be considered zoonotic or potentially zoonotic. *Salmonellae* have several virulence factors that contribute to clinical symptoms

[a] Exotics Medicine Service, Centre Hospitalier Universitaire d'Alfort, Ecole Nationale Vétérinaire d'Alfort, 7 Avenue du Général de Gaulle, 94700 Maisons-Alfort, France
[b] Department of Small Animal Medicine & Surgery, College of Veterinary Medicine, University of Georgia, 501 DW Brooks Drive, Athens, GA 30602, USA
* Corresponding author.
E-mail address: cppignon@vet-alfort.fr

Vet Clin Exot Anim 14 (2011) 533–549
doi:10.1016/j.cvex.2011.05.004
1094-9194/11/$ – see front matter © 2011 Elsevier Inc. All rights reserved.

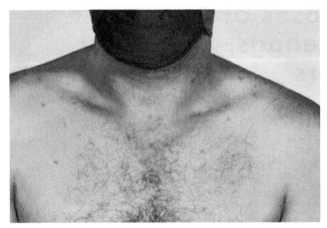

Fig. 1. Rose spots indicative of systemic infection on the chest of a patient with typhoid fever from *Salmonella typhi*. Although *S typhi* is not zoonotic, similar symptoms can occur in severe infections with other *Salmonella* serotypes. (*Courtesy of* Centers for Disease Control and Prevention Public Health Image Library; available at: http://phil.cdc.gov/phil/home.asp.)

including diarrhea, bacteremia, and septicemia. These factors include the lipopolysaccharide of the outer wall, pili, flagella, cytotoxin, and enterotoxin.[1]

Salmonellosis occurs worldwide. *S enteritidis* is the most prevalent causative serotype, followed by *S typhimurium*. Changes in the relative frequency of serotypes can be observed over short periods of time, sometimes within 1 or 2 years. Only a limited number of serotypes are typically isolated from man or animals in a single region or country.

Salmonellosis is perhaps the most widespread zoonosis in the world[2] and occurs both in sporadic cases and outbreaks affecting a family or several hundreds to thousands of people. The true incidence is difficult to evaluate because many countries do not have an epidemiologic surveillance system in place[3]; however, the US Centers for Disease Control and Prevention estimates that approximately 1.4 million cases occur in the United States annually.

Salmonellae of animal origin cause an intestinal infection in man characterized by a 6- to 72-hour incubation period after ingestion of the implicated food, followed by a sudden onset of fever, myalgias, headache, and malaise. The main symptoms consist of abdominal pain, nausea, vomiting, and diarrhea. In some cases, patients have a rash of flat, red spots indicating systemic infection (**Fig. 1**); Reiter syndrome, a reactive arthritis, can also occur in some cases. Salmonellosis normally has a benign course and clinical recovery ensues in 2 to 4 days with rehydration and electrolyte replacement. Although salmonellosis may occur in persons of all ages, the prevalence is higher among children and the elderly. A high proportion of *Salmonella* strains with resistance to multiple antibiotics have been seen in many countries.[4]

In pets, *Salmonellae* have a wide variety of domestic and wild animal hosts. The rate of infection in domestic animals has been estimated to be 1% to 3%,[5] and some reports indicate that salmonellosis occurs less frequently in pets.[6] Infection may or may not be clinically apparent. In the subclinical form, an animal may have a latent infection and harbor the pathogen in lymph nodes, or it may be a carrier and shed the organism in fecal material either briefly, intermittently, or persistently.[6]

Ferrets

Clinical signs of salmonellosis in ferrets include conjunctivitis, anorexia, lethargy, vomiting, fever, dehydration, abdominal pain, diarrhea with or without blood, tenesmus, mesenteric lymphadenopathy, weight loss, and pale mucus membranes.[5,7–9] With septicemia and septic shock, there may be evidence of weakness, cardiovascular collapse, and disseminated intravascular coagulation.[7,10]

Successful treatment of infected ferrets requires aggressive supportive care, including appropriate fluid therapy and nutritional support.[7,8,10] Hypoglycemia is common with sepsis and must be recognized immediately and corrected.[11] *Salmonella spp* isolated from ferrets have shown resistance to several antibiotics; therefore, antimicrobial selection should be based on culture and sensitivity testing.[9,10] The use of antibiotics can be controversial, but suggested antibiotics include trimethoprim-sulfamethoxazole, enrofloxacin, and chloramphenicol.[7,12]

Both clinically ill ferrets and asymptomatic carriers may serve as primary sources of infection to humans.[7,10] Clients should be advised to avoid feeding raw meat and poultry products to ferrets and to follow sound hygiene practices.[9] As raw food and whole prey diets for pets increase in popularity, salmonellosis should always be suspected in cases of diarrhea and septicemia in ferrets. Diagnosis of animal salmonellosis is made by culturing *Salmonella spp* from fecal material, but selective media such as xylose-lysine-desoxycholate agar are required for isolation.[5,7,9] Sampling of fecal samples over several days may improve the chances of isolating the organism.[8]

Hedgehogs

Several serotypes of *Salmonella* occur in hedgehogs, and cases of transmission from pet African hedgehogs to humans have been documented.[13–16] *Salmonella* serotype *Tilene* has been isolated from an African pygmy hedgehog and associated with clinical disease in a 10-year-old child.[17]

Hedgehogs have soft droppings and a propensity to walk in their feces, which may facilitate dissemination of *Salmonella* throughout the household. As with reptiles, it should be assumed that all pet hedgehogs can carry and transmit this pathogen. Subclinically infected animals may shed the organism intermittently; therefore, negative fecal cultures should not be used to rule out the carrier state. Treatment to eliminate the carrier state in an animal is unlikely to be successful and should not be attempted because antibiotic resistance may result.

Sugar gliders

Few reports of laboratory-confirmed cases of human salmonellosis associated with exposure to sugar gliders have been described.[18,19]

Transmission and prevention

Humans and animals become infected with *Salmonella* by ingestion of the organism, most often by consumption of fecally contaminated food. Numerous animals can act as reservoirs of zoonotic *Salmonellae,* and the most common foods associated with human infection are contaminated poultry, pork, beef, eggs, milk, and milk and egg products.[20,21] Humans can also contract the infection directly from contact with domestic animals or house pets[22]; animals can have fecal contamination on their coats, which can be ingested by the care taker after handling. Humans should always wash their hands after handling an animal to reduce the risk of ingestion of the organism. Additionally, animals and their enclosures should not be cleaned in the kitchen to reduce the likelihood of contaminating cooking surfaces and utensils with infected feces.

Campylobacteriosis

Campylobacter jejuni and occasionally *C coli* are responsible for human infections. *C jejuni* is a gram-negative, slender, microaerophilic, spiral to curved bacterial rod[10,23] and has a characteristic darting or corkscrew motion.[9,23] Campylobacteriosis has a worldwide distribution.

At present, *C jejuni* is among the principal bacterial agents that causes enteritis and diarrhea in humans, particularly in developed countries. In developed countries, the incidence of campylobacteriosis is similar to that of enteritis caused by *Salmonella,* and according to Benenson,[24] *Campylobacter* causes 5% to 14% of diarrhea cases worldwide.

Enteritis caused by *C jejuni* is an acute illness with an incubation period of 2 to 5 days. The principal symptoms are diarrhea, fever, abdominal pain, vomiting in one third of patients, and visible or occult blood in the feces of 50% to 90% of patients. Fever is often accompanied by general malaise, headache, and muscle and joint pain. The course of the illness is usually self-limiting, and the patient recovers spontaneously in 7 to 10 days; acute symptoms often fade in 2 to 3 days. Symptoms may be more severe in some patients and are similar to those of ulcerative colitis and salmonellosis. Complications are rare and include meningitis, Guillain-Barre syndrome, and spontaneous abortions. Enteric campylobacteriosis does not usually require medication, but electrolyte and fluid replacement is often needed. As with salmonellosis, antibiotic use is controversial because of the development of antibiotic-resistant strains; however, when warranted, erythromycin is the antibiotic of choice; enrofloxacin-resistant strains of *C jejuni* have been identified and use of enrofloxacin in poultry is banned.

Domestic and wild mammals and birds are the main reservoirs of *C jejuni*, but it can be difficult to implicate this agent as a cause of diarrheal disease because of the high prevalence of asymptomatic infections in animals. *C jejuni* can be isolated from the feces of clinically normal ferrets,[7,9,10,23] but is not usually a cause of primary gastrointestinal disease in this species. *C coli* was isolated from the intestines of a 16-week-old female ferret in a group of ferrets housed at a commercial ferret farm; the animal showed clinical signs including anorexia, weight loss, and diarrhea.[25] To the authors' knowledge, there is no report of campylobacteriosis in hedgehogs or sugar gliders.

Affected ferrets can develop a self-limiting diarrhea, and clinical signs occur more often in ferrets less than 6 months of age.[10] The diarrhea can contain mucous and be watery or bile streaked, with or without blood and leukocytes.[7,10,26] Anorexia, fever, dehydration, and tenesmus can also be observed.[7,14,10] Stress and concurrent illness may increase the likelihood of clinical disease.[7,10] Rectal prolapses in mink (*Mustela vison*) kits have been observed in natural and experimental infections with *C jejuni*.[10] Experimental infection in pregnant ferrets led to abortion, and *C jejuni* was isolated from the uterine contents of 2 jills.[27]

Campylobacter spp may be detected in gram-stained feces or through fecal wet mount evaluation using a high phase or dark field objective.[7] Definitive diagnosis requires bacterial culture on selective media, but these bacteria can be difficult to grow and false-negative results are common.[7,10,23] The organism can also be identified by polymerase chain reaction (PCR) using primers to the 16S rDNA.[7,23]

Although erythromycin has been shown to clear *C jejuni* from fecal samples in humans, experimental administration in ferrets (40 mg/kg twice a day for 5 days) did not eliminate the carrier state in 1 study.[12] The authors of this study postulated that treatment failure was because of inadequate dosage or frequency of drug delivery or through reinfection.[12] Other suggested drug protocols are available in the litera-ture.[7,12] The isolation of *C jejuni* from asymptomatic ferrets and the fact that *Campylobacter spp* are a known cause of enteritis in humans suggests a risk for zoonotic transmission.[9]

Transmission occurs through ingestion of and direct contact with feces or contaminated water or foods, such as uncooked poultry.[7,9,10] The organism is capable of surviving freezing and has been shown to survive for several months in frozen poultry, minced meat, and certain chilled foods. Infected dogs and cats, and potentially ferrets, may transmit the organism to humans.[23] Prevention measures are similar to those previously described for *Salmonella*.

Mycobacteriosis

Mycobacteria are aerobic bacilli found in a variety of animal species, including humans, and also live freely in the environment. They are intracellular dwelling and capable of developing resistance to a variety of antimicrobial agents.[9,23] The most significant members of the genera in terms of possible zoonotic infections are *M bovis* (found in cattle, dogs and pigs), *M avium* (found in birds, pigs, and sheep), and *M marinum* (found in seals, sea lions, and fish).[28] The distribution of *M bovis* and *M tuberculosis* is worldwide.

Infection usually starts with the development of foci in either the lungs or the gastrointestinal tract, but cutaneous inoculation can also occur. Disseminated infec-tion may develop from these foci, with an associated morbidity and mortality, especially in cases of advanced HIV infection. After infection, there can be a short or long incubation period depending on the health of the individual and the strain and virulence of the organism. The disease progresses with the organism becoming disseminated throughout the body, and sites of colonization are usually the lungs, lymph nodes, circulatory system, the liver, spleen, and other major organs. Symptoms vary depending on the sites of infection and can include loss of appetite, anorexia, intermittent fever, weariness, and extreme fatigue. The disease can also manifest as a cutaneous form with ulcers and lesions that progress to persistent suppurative sores.[29]

Ferrets

Ferrets may be naturally or experimentally affected by *M bovis*, *M avium*, and *M tuberculosis*.[30] *M bovis* and *M avium* infections have been recognized in research and farm ferrets in England, Europe, and New Zealand.[31–34] These infections may have been associated with the feeding of raw meat and poultry and unpasteurized dairy products. More recently, a pet ferret was reported to have a visceral infection caused by *M avium*.[34] The ferret had a long-term history of weight loss, diarrhea, and vomiting that was unresponsive to treatment. *Mycobacteria* have also been isolated from the gastrointestinal tract of ferrets and infection is characterized by a disseminated gastric lesion produced by *M celatum* (type 3). Clinical signs in infected ferrets can include enlarged lymph nodes, organomegaly (liver), unthrifty condition, weight loss despite a normal appetite, elevated white blood count, elevated liver enzyme activity, and diarrhea; clinical signs vary based on the location of the granulomas. Granulo-matous enteritis can produce vomiting, anorexia, and diarrhea in the affected ferret.[11]

Hedgehogs

Systemic mycobacteriosis caused by *M marinum* has been reported in pet European hedgehogs.[35] A European hedgehog was brought for treatment of nonsuppurative masses in the subcutis of the ventral cervical region.[35] The animal worsened and died. On necropsy, multiple granulomatous lesions found in the lymph nodes, lungs, spleen, liver, and heart were positive for *M marinum* in culture. In the reported case, the hedgehog apparently acquired *M marinum* from the fish tank in which the animal was housed at a pet store.[35] In humans, the organism is associated with a cutaneous disease of the extremities (arms) called "fish-tank granuloma," which is typically contracted from contact with aquariums.[36] The organism typically gains entry through a wound or abrasion in the skin, such as may be produced by hedgehog spines, and can spread systemically along the lymphatic system. The resulting disease produces lesions resembling those of sporotrichosis, tularemia, nocardiosis, and blastomycosis.[36]

Skin testing is often used for diagnosis in humans, but false-negative and –positive results can occur because of exposure to different *Mycobacterium* species; skin testing has not been evaluated for diagnosis in ferrets, hedgehogs, or sugar gliders. Isolation and culture are difficult owing to the intracellular nature and slow growth of the bacterium; however, this does produce a definitive diagnosis and also allows for drug-sensitivity testing. Intestinal biopsy results can reveal granulomatous inflammation and acid-fast bacteria; acid-fast staining, PCR testing, and culture can aid in diagnosis.

Because of it zoonotic potential, treatment of mycobacteriosis is not recommended. If owners insist on pursuing treatment for an infected animal, a waiver explaining the risks of the organism to people should be signed by the owner. Multidrug protocols are typically required because *Mycobacteria* routinely develop resistance.

Transmission and prevention

In general, *Mycobacteria* are transmitted from infected individuals, either humans or animals, primarily via aerosols. Infection is also possible via contact with or ingestion of infected tissue, bodily secretions, or body fluids such as milk, blood, or plasma. Cutaneous inoculation is also possible via bites, cuts, or lacerations[37]; exposure from hedgehogs would most likely occur from cutaneous inoculation after an injury from the spines. Preventive measures include euthanizing confirmed *Mycobacterium*-positive animals, washing hands after handling an animal, wearing disposable gloves and masks when handling sick animals, and wearing protective gloves when handling hedgehogs.

Other Bacteria

Yersiniae are facultatively anaerobic, gram-negative rods and members of the family Enterobacteriaceae.[23] *Y pestis* is the causative agent of bubonic plague and resembles a safety pin when stained with Wright, Giemsa, or Wayson stains.[23] The life cycle generally is flea–rodent–flea, with occasional breakouts to other species.[23] Infection in carnivores typically occurs through ingestion of infected prey, although transmission by a flea bite is also possible. There are no published reports of clinical disease in the domestic ferret, although ferrets are susceptible to infestation by dog and cat fleas. Clinical disease has been reported in black footed ferrets (*Mustela nigripes*).[38–40] *Y pestis* was isolated from an endemic hedgehog in Madagascar, but no reports of the disease in pet hedgehogs are in the literature. The plague can be treated with antibiotics and can be prevented by keeping pets inside and maintaining appropriate flea control.

Y pseudotuberculosis has been isolated in the United Kingdom from 2 wild hedgehogs that died at a rehabilitation center in Berkshire.[41] In humans, the organism primarily causes a gastroenteritis characterized by a self-limiting mesenteric lymphadenitis that mimics appendicitis. Postinfectious complications include erythema nodosum and reactive arthritis[42]; however, no reports of transmission to humans from ferrets, hedgehogs, or sugar gliders are found in the literature.

Leptospira grippotyphosa and *L icterohaemorrhagiae* have been isolated from asymptomatic ferrets, although reports in this species are fragmentary at best.[43] Historically, ferrets were used to control rodent populations and could easily have been exposed to leptospires in rodent urine.[43] Ferrets raised in the fur industry have also contracted leptospirosis, and pet ferrets exposed to infected dogs may be at risk for contracting the disease. In New Zealand, despite having a high prevalence of infection in mice and rats commonly eaten by free-living ferrets, no animals had serologic evidence of infection and culture of renal tissues was negative in 1 study.[44] There is no evidence today of transmission of leptospirosis from a ferret to a human.

FUNGAL ZOONOSES
Dermatophytosis

Several species of *Microsporum*, *Trichophyton*, and *Epidermophyton floccosum* are known to cause dermatophytosis. Ecologically and epidemiologically, 3 groups of species are distinguished according to the reservoir: Anthropophilic, zoophilic, and geophilic. This discussion considers only zoophilic species transmissible to man. The most important zoophilic species are *M canis, T mentagrophytes (Arthroderma benhamiae)*, and *T verrucosum*.

Among the zoophilic species, *M canis, T verrucosum, T equinum*, and *T mentagrophytes* are distributed worldwide. *T mentagrophytes var. erinacei* has limited distribution (France, Great Britain, Italy, and New Zealand) and *T simii* is limited to Asia.

Dermatophytic infections are common, but the exact prevalence is unknown. The disease is not notifiable; moreover, many people with minor infections do not seek medical treatment. A retrospective study of 1717 Ministry of Agriculture veterinarians in the United Kingdom found that dermatophytosis was the most common zoonosis, with a prevalence of 24%.[45]

Dermatophytosis is a superficial infection of the keratinized parts of the body (skin, hair, and nails). The *Microsporum* species cause most cases of tinea capitis and tinea corporis, and the *Trichophyton* species can affect the skin at any part of the body. Transmission from animal to man is probably caused by contact with hair from infected animals. Currently, *M canis* is among the principal etiologic agents of tinea, and the incubation period is 1 to 2 weeks. Tinea of the scalp is most frequent among children aged 4 to 11 years and its incidence is greater among boys. The disease begins with a small papule, the hair becomes brittle, and the infection spreads peripherally, leaving scaly, bald patches. Suppurative lesions (kerions) are frequent when the fungus is of animal origin. Tinea caused by *M canis* heals spontaneously during puberty.

Tinea corporis (**Fig. 2**) is characterized by flat lesions that tend to be annular. The borders are reddish and may be raised, with microvesicles or scales. Tinea corporis in children is usually an extension of tinea capitis to the face and is typically caused by *M canis* or *M audouinii*. Active lesions may also occur on the wrists and neck of mothers or young adults who have contact with an infected child. Tinea corporis in adults, occurring primarily on the limbs and torso, is chronic in nature and usually is caused by the anthropophilic dermatophyte *T rubrum*.[46]

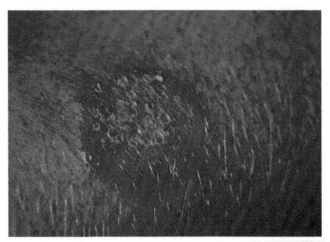

Fig. 2. Patient presented with ringworm, or tinea corporis, on the arm from *Trichophyton mentagrophytes.* The genus *Trichophyton* inhabits the soil, humans or animals, and is among the leading causes of hair, skin, and nail infections, or dermatophytosis in humans. (*Courtesy of* Centers for Disease Control and Prevention Public Health Image Library; available at: http://phil.cdc.gov/phil/home.asp.)

Ferrets

Dermatophytosis is rare in ferrets; however, when it occurs is usually caused by either *M canis* or *T mentagrophytes.*[47–54] Young and immunosuppressed animals are most susceptible to developing infection. Cohabiting cats may be the source of infection. Clinical lesions are typically cutaneous, and include areas of annular alopecia, broken hairs, diffuse scaling, erythema, and crusting. Pruritus is not normally seen.[50,54]

Diagnosis is made on the basis of microscopic examination of affected hairs. Skin scrapes and hair samples may be submitted for fungal culture. Some isolates of *M canis* may fluoresce, but a negative Woods lamp test should not exclude dermatophytosis as a possible diagnosis. Spontaneous remission has been reported.[48,55] Treatments for dermatophytosis in ferrets have been published, and treatment should be administered for 1 month past resolution of clinical signs. Environmental disinfection is important for prevention. Bleach diluted 1:1 with warm water can be used to clean the environment and cages; caging and accessories should be well rinsed and aired before animals are allowed contact with them. For now, there is no confirmed case of transmission from a ferret to a person, although the potential does exist.

Hedgehogs

Dermatophytosis in the hedgehog is usually caused by *T erinacei* (*T mentagrophytes var. erinacei*), but can occasionally be caused by *Microsporum canis* and *M gypseum.* Several cases of human dermatophytosis transmitted from pet hedgehogs have been documented.[56] Details are given of 5 cases of human infection with *T mentagrophytes var. erinacei* [*T erinacei*]. *T erinacei* was isolated from 47 (11.5%) of 408 healthy hedgehogs and from 4 of 5 with skin lesions.

Transmission in hedgehogs is probably by direct contact from mother to young or during fights or courtship, which may explain why most lesions are on the head. Infection may also be obtained from environmental spores, which can remain viable in dry nests for up to 1 year. Clinical signs are typically located around the head and include crusting lesions around the base of spines and hair and spine loss. Bleeding may occur if the scabs are removed. Thickening of the pinnae may also occur in chronic infections. Pruritus and debility is generally absent, even with severe infections, with affected animals gaining weight normally.[57]

Definitive diagnosis is by fungal culture. The necessity for treatment is debatable, given the low pathogenicity of infection and its widespread nature, but the zoonotic potential may provide justification. Recovery and spine regrowth can take up to 1 month. Infection in humans can be prevented by wearing gardening gloves when handling hedgehogs and washing hands and forearms with soap and water after handling an infected animal.

Other Fungal Zoonoses

Blastomycosis[58] and coccidiomycosis[59] are 2 potential zoonotic diseases that have been reported in ferrets; however, there are no published cases documenting transmission from a ferret to a human.

VIRAL ZOONOSES
Influenza

Influenza viruses have an RNA genome and are of the family Orthomyxoviridae. Four types are recognized: A, B, C, and thogotovirus. The surface antigens are of particular immunologic and epidemiologic interest. These antigens, which reside in protein subunits on the viral envelope, are hemagglutinin (H) and neuraminidase (N). Fourteen hemagglutinin antigens (H1–H14) and 9 neuraminidase antigens (N1–N9) are recognized.[59] The influenza A viruses infect a large variety of animals, as well as humans. There is less certainty about influenza types B and C, and thogotovirus in animals. Influenza viruses occur worldwide.

Influenza usually occurs as an annual epidemic and is characterized by high morbidity and low mortality. Pandemics have occurred at irregular intervals (from 9 to 39 years) and have been due to major changes in the genes that code the H and N antigens.[59] Type A influenza occurs especially in swine, equines, cats, seals, ferrets, minks, and numerous wild and domestic avian species.[59]

The incubation period of influenza viruses is 1 to 3 days, and disease has a sudden onset with fever, chills, cephalalgia, myalgia, fatigue, and sometimes prostration. Other common symptoms are conjunctival inflammation, intense lacrimation, nonproductive coughing, sneezing, runny nose, sore throat, and painful swallowing. Approximately 20% of patients have rales, but this does not necessarily indicate pulmonary involvement.[59] The disease has a rapid course, with recovery in about 7 days.

Ferrets

Human influenza types A and B are pathogenic to ferrets.[59] Ferrets also are susceptible to avian, seal, equine, and swine influenza A viruses, although only human, avian, and swine strains induce clinical signs.[60–64] Ferrets became ill after exposure to the pandemic H1N1 influenza virus.[65] Infection with influenza B virus less frequently results in illness and is associated with a milder clinical course.[59] Transmission of influenza virus from human to ferrets and vice versa was documented in the 1930s.[66,67] Ferrets are used extensively as an animal model for influenza virus pathogenesis and immunity studies because their biologic response to influenza infection is similar to that of humans.[68,69]

Influenza virus is transmitted by aerosol droplets from an infected individual, either to a human or a ferret. After intranasal inoculation, the virus localizes and replicates in the nasal mucosa.[70] After a short incubation period, the body temperature increases and then decreases approximately 48 hours later.[71] Transmission of the virus begins at the height of pyrexia and continues for 3 to 4 days.[68]

As in humans, the disease is characterized by upper respiratory signs. Clinical signs appear 48 hours postinfection and include anorexia, malaise, fever, sneezing, and serous nasal discharge.[59,71] Infection usually is mild in adult ferrets compared with neonates, who can become severely ill.[72] Conjunctivitis, photosensitivity, and unilateral otitis also may be seen.[59,73] Influenza infection may involve the lower respiratory tract in some animals[59,74]; however, influenza virus is usually confined to the bronchial and bronchiolar tissues.[68,75] The disease may be fatal in 1- to 2-day-old ferret kits secondary to bronchiolitis, pneumonia, and aspiration of material from the upper respiratory tract.[72,76,77] Clinical signs of influenza can be similar to those of distemper in ferrets.

Generally, the diagnosis of influenza infection is based on the presence of compatible clinical signs, a history of exposure to infected individuals, and recovery from illness within 7 to 10 days. The use of virus isolation or hemagglutinin-inhibiting antibody titers on acute and convalescent serum samples rarely is needed for diagnosis.[59] An enzyme-linked immunosorbent assay has been used to detect antibodies against influenza A and may be used to obtain a diagnosis rapidly.[78]

Treatments to relieve clinical symptoms should be used on a case-by-case basis. Antibiotics may be indicated to control secondary bacterial infections of the respiratory tract and reduce mortality[79]; neonates are especially susceptible to secondary bacterial infections. Administration of antiviral medication has been studied in humans and ferrets, but use is controversial owing to the development of resistant strains.

Vaccination of ferrets against influenza virus generally is not recommended because it is usually a mild disease and the antigenic variation of the virus complicates vaccination[59,63]; however, vaccination of humans for seasonal influenza and H1N1 is currently recommended. Controlling influenza infection resides in avoiding exposure to infected individuals, either ferret or human. Owners should be advised to minimize contact with their ferrets if they or the ferret have a respiratory infection and should be sure to wash their hands thoroughly before changing the animal's cage, food, and water; masks can also be worn to reduce respiratory transmission. Veterinarians with respiratory infections should consider wearing a mask and gloves.

Foot and Mouth Virus

The foot-and-mouth disease virus is a picornavirus, a member of the Aphthovirus genus in the Picornaviridae family. Hedgehogs are susceptible to foot-and-mouth disease and can act as carriers of the virus.[80,81] It is unclear whether they act as a reservoir for the disease. Early studies indicating latent infection should be viewed with caution because the virologic techniques used at the time were unreliable and there is little evidence that hedgehogs have been involved in the spread of foot-and-mouth disease in Europe or Africa.[81] Affected animals show vesicles, erythema, and swelling on the haired parts of the body, the feet, lips, and perineum.[81] Anorexia, sneezing, and hypersalivation are also prominent clinical signs. Diagnosis is made on the presence of clinical signs and viral isolation, and treatment is not normally undertaken.

This disease can be transmitted to humans, who can be asymptomatic carriers and shed the virus for a long period; the virus presents a far greater threat to hoofstock. Importation of African hedgehogs has been banned by the US Department of

Agriculture since 1991 to prevent introduction of the disease. The current pet trade in the United States consists entirely of captive-bred animals.

PARASITIC ZOONOSES
Scabies

The agent of human scabies is *Sarcoptes scabiei var hominis*, an oval mite. This species has varieties that infest approximately 40 species of mammals, from primates to marsupials.[82] Each variety is strongly host specific, although some can infest other species and cause temporary illness.

Sarcoptes is distributed worldwide. Human scabies is prevalent primarily among socioeconomic classes whose members are poor, often malnourished, and have inadequate hygiene; overcrowding promotes the spread of the mite and poor hygiene is conducive to its persistence.[83] Zoonotic scabies infections are typically mild and the most prominent symptom is itching, which is especially intense at night, forcing patients to scratch themselves. Scratching can cause lesions, new foci of scabies, and, often, purulent secondary infections. It is believed that animal mites do not generally excavate tunnels in human skin and that the infestation is more superficial and self-limiting. An infestation that lasts longer is usually due to ongoing exposure and permanent superinfestation. Treatment of the animal with scabies is usually sufficient to eliminate human zoonotic scabies without treatment.

Ferrets

S scabiei is the cause of sarcoptic mange in ferrets, but its occurrence is rare, especially among animals kept indoors.[84,85] Dogs can act as a source of contagion for ferrets.[84,86] Mites burrow in tunnels in the skin, especially in sites that are poorly haired. In severe cases, extensive areas can be affected. *S scabiei* generalized alopecia, intense pruritus, or localized lesions of the toes and feet. Lesions are particularly prominent on sparsely haired sites. The skin becomes alopecic and lichenified with associated exudation and crusting. Nails can become deformed and slough.[84,86–88] Diagnosis is by skin scrapings, although false-negative results are common[85,89]; treatments for ferrets have been published. Affected and in-contact animals should be treated and the environment and caging thoroughly cleaned.[85,87–89]

Hedgehogs

Sarcoptes spp. is occasionally seen in young hedgehogs.[90–93] This parasite can cause generalized erythema, alopecia, and quill loss, and can be fatal. Diagnosis is made by identification of mites on scrapings from the skin. Therapy can be undertaken using ivermectin.

Sarcoptes is mainly transmitted by recently inseminated female mites before they begin to build their tunnels.[83] The skin of the susceptible individual must be in close contact with the skin of the infested individual. In the case of interhuman transmission of *Sarcoptes*, the mite has been found on fomites, and thus contagion through contaminated objects may be possible. Because the parasite can survive for several days off an animal's body on clothing, towels, bedclothes, and other items, these objects can serve as sources of infection. Each animal species is a reservoir of the mite that attacks its own kind, but cross-transmission between species occasionally occurs. Zoonotic scabies does occur, but is a minor public health problem because it typically resolves spontaneously and is not transmitted between humans. Infected animals should be treated and housing should be cleaned and disinfected to prevent transmission to humans.

Cryptosporidiosis and Giardiasis

Cryptosporidium are protozoa of the coccidia group in the phylum *Apicomplexa* (formerly Sporozoa).[83] The only specie that affects both humans and other mammals is *Cryptosporidum parvum*.[94] *C parvum* normally lives in the small intestine, where it forms oocysts that are excreted in the host's feces. Distribution of *C parvum* is worldwide. Cases of human cryptosporidiosis have been reported from greater than 50 countries on 6 continents.[95] The illness in humans is characterized by profuse watery diarrhea, which begins 1 to 2 weeks after infection and generally lasts 8 to 20 days, often accompanied by abdominal pain, nausea, vomiting, low-grade fever (<102°F; <39°C), and weight loss. In immunodeficient individuals, the symptoms are more severe, and the parasite has sometimes been found to invade the respiratory and biliary tracts.[96]

Young ferrets can be infected with *C parvum*, but the disease is usually self-limiting and subclinical, even in animals experimentally immunosuppressed.[85,86] Recent studies in genetic sequencing have shown that the ferret genotype of *C parvum* is unique, but the zoonotic potential is not known.[85,97] Intestinal cryptosporidiosis has been described in a captive juvenile African pygmy hedgehog.[98] Large numbers of *Cryptosporidium* spp. developmental stages were present throughout much of the affected animal's intestine. The protozoan in this report was not identified to species, but zoonotic potential exists and appropriate precautions should be taken to prevent transmission to humans.[98] Control of infection is through elimination of infective oocysts in the environment and avoidance of contact with known sources of infection including contaminated food or water sources.[86] Isolates of *Cryptosporidium* should be considered potentially zoonotic until more data are available, and infected ferrets should be isolated from children and immunosuppressed individuals.[85,86,99]

G intestinalis is a flagellate protozoan whose life cycle includes trophozoites in the vegetative stage and cysts in the transmission stage; the taxonomy of the species of the genus *Giardia* is still controversial. Three morphologic forms are currently accepted: *G intestinalis*, which affects man, domestic animals, and other mammals; *G muris*, which affects birds, rodents, and reptiles; and *G agilis*, which affects amphibians.[100] Transmission is fecal–oral after the passage of cysts in the feces of an infected animal. The majority of infections in humans are subclinical.[101] In symptomatic individuals, the incubation period is generally 3 to 25 days[101] and symptoms consist mainly of diarrhea and bloating, frequently accompanied by abdominal pain. Nausea and vomiting occur less frequently. The acute phase of the disease lasts 3 to 4 days. In some persons, giardiasis may be a prolonged illness, with episodes of recurring diarrhea and flatulence, urticaria, and intolerance of certain foods.

Clinical reports of giardiasis in the domestic ferret are scarce[84,85,102]; dogs and cats may serve as reservoirs of infection to ferrets.[84] In 1 report,[103] *G intestinalis* was isolated from an asymptomatic ferret housed at a pet store. This *Giardia* isolate was determined through genetic analysis to be in genetic group A-I, which may have zoonotic potential.[103] Debilitated ferrets, or those that have concurrent disease, are more likely to shed *Giardia spp.*[84] *Giardia* has been reported as a suspected agent of chronic diarrhea in sugar gliders.[104]

Because the oocysts of *C parvum* and the cysts of *G intestinalis* can live for long periods in water, public water supplies should be protected against contamination by human and animal fecal matter. Adequate systems of sedimentation, flocculation, and filtration can remove *Cryptosporidium* and *Giardia* from water, allowing the use of surface water supply systems. Personal hygiene is essential, and includes handwashing and not eating while handling potentially infected animals. Individual prevention measures include boiling or filtering suspicious water or drinking bottled water. Fecal matter should be disposed of in a manner that will not contaminate drinking water systems. Although there are no data describing the prevalence of transmission from pets to human, animals with potentially zoonotic cryptosporidiosis or giardiasis should be treated when appropriate because they may frequently come into contact with children.[105]

SUMMARY

Multiple zoonoses are described in exotics species. For some of these zoonoses, we have proof of transmission to human, but in other cases the potential for transmission is real because the same pathogen can induce clinical signs in humans and in animals. Zoonoses should be understood and recognized because, as veterinarians, it is our duty to care for animals and educate owners and staff to prevent disease.

REFERENCES

1. Murray MJ. Salmonella: virulence factors and enteric salmonellosis. J Am Vet Med Assoc 1986;189:145–7.
2. Rodrigue DC, Tauxe RV, Rowe B. International increase in Salmonella enteritidis: a new pandemic? Epidemiol Infect 1990;105:21–7.
3. Hargrett-Bean NT, Pavia AT, Tauxe TV. Salmonella isolates from humans in the United States, 1984–1986. MMWR Morb Mortal Wkly Rep 1988;37(Suppl 2):25–31.
4. Van den Bogaard AE, Stobberingh EE. Epidemiology of resistance to antibiotics: links between animals and humans. Int J Antimicrob Agents 2000;14:327–35.
5. United States of America, Department of Health and Human Services, Centers for Disease Control and Prevention (CDC). Salmonella surveillance. Annual summary 1980. Atlanta: CDC; 1982.
6. Zoonoses and communicable diseases common to man and animals, vol. I: bacteriose and mycoses. 3rd edition. Washington (DC): Pan American Health Organization; 2001.
7. Oglesbee BL. The 5-minute veterinary consult: ferret and rabbit. Ames (IA): Blackwell Publishing; 2006.
8. Hoefer HL, Bell JA. Gastrointestinal diseases. In: Carpenter JW, Quesenberry KE, editors. Ferrets, rabbits, and rodents: clinical medicine and surgery. 2nd edition. St. Louis: Saunders; 2000. p. 25–40.
9. Marini RP, Otto G, Erdman S, et al. Biology and diseases of ferrets. In: Fox JG, Anderson LC, Loew FM, et al, editors. Laboratory animal medicine. 2nd edition. Amsterdam: Academic Press; 2002. p. 483–517.
10. Fox JG. Bacterial and mycoplasmal diseases. In: Fox JG, editor. Biology and diseases of the ferret. 2nd edition. Baltimore: Williams & Wilkins; 1998. p. 321–54.
11. Valheim M, Djonne B, Heiene R, et al. Disseminated *Mycobacterium celatum* (type 3) infection in a domestic ferret (Mustela putorius furo). Vet Pathol 2001;38:460–3.
12. Fox JG, Moore R, Ackerman JI. Canine and feline campylobacteriosis: epizootiology and clinical and public health features. J Am Vet Med Assoc 1983;183:1420–4.
13. Woodward D, Khakhria R, Johnson W. Human salmonellosis associated with exotic pets. J Clin Microbiol 1997;35:2786–90.
14. US Centers for Disease Control and Prevention. African pygmy hedgehog-associated salmonellosis—Washington, 1994. MMWR Morb Mortal Wkly Rep 1995;44: 462–3.

15. Isenbugel E, Baumgartner R. Diseases of the hedgehog. In: Fowler M, editor. Zoo and wild animal medicine 3rd edition. Philadelphia: WB Saunders Company; 1993.
16. Craig C, Styliadis S, Woodward D, Werker D. African pygmy hedgehog-associated Salmonella tilene in Canada. Can Commun Dis Rep 1997;23:1292.
17. US Centers for Disease Control and Prevention (CDC). African pygmy hedgehog associated salmonellosis—Washington, 1994. MMWR Morb Mortal Wkly Rep 1995; 44:462–3.
18. Woodward DL, Khakhria R, Johnson WM. Human salmonellosis associated with exotic pets. Journal of Clinical Microbiology 1997;35:2786–90.
19. Johnson-Delaney CA. Marsupial medicine and surgery. Proceeding of the 80th Western Veterinary Conference. Las Vegas (NV); 1997.
20. Aoust D. Salmonella. In: Doyle MP, editor. Foodborne bacterial pathogens. New York: Marcel Dekker; 1989.
21. Stevens A, Joseph C, Bruce J, et al. A large outbreak of Salmonella enteritidis phage type 4 associated with eggs from overseas. Epidemiol Infect 1989;103:425–33.
22. World Health Organization (WHO) Expert Committee on Salmonellosis Control. Salmonellosis Control. The role of animal and product hygiene (Technical Report Series 774). Report of a WHO Expert Committee. Geneva (Switzerland): WHO; 1988.
23. Songer JG, Post KW. Veterinary microbiology: bacterial and fungal agents of animal disease. St. Louis: Saunders; 2005. p. 95–109.
24. Benenson AS, editor. Control of communicable diseases in man. 15th edition. An official report of the American Public Health Association. Washington (DC): American Public Health Association; 1990.
25. Larson DJ, Hoffman LJ. Isolation of *Campylobacter coli* from a proliferative intestinal lesion in a ferret. J Vet Diagn Invest 1990;2:238–9.
26. Bell JA, Manning DD. Pathogenicity of *Campylobacter jejuni* in intraperitoneally or intravenously inoculated ferrets. Curr Microbiol 1990;21:47–51.
27. Bell JA, Manning DD. Reproductive failure in mink and ferrets after intravenous or oral inoculation of *Campylobacter jejuni*. Can J Vet Res 1990;54:432–7.
28. Adams R, Remington J, Steinberg J, et al. Fish aquariums a source of *Mycobacterium marinum* infections resembling sporotrichosis. JAMA 1970;211:457–61.
29. Wolinsky E. Nontuberculous mycobacteria and associated diseases. Am Rev Resp Dis 1979;119:107–59.
30. A chronic granulomatous intestinal disease in ferret caused by an acid fast organism Bryant Lab Animal Science 1988;38:498–9.
31. Valheim M, Djonne B, Heiene R, et al. Disseminated *Mycobacterium celatum* (type 3) infection in a domestic ferret (*Mustela putorius furo*). Vet Pathol 2001;38:460–3.
32. de Lisle GW, Kawakami RP, Yates GF, et al. Isolation of *Mycobacterium bovis* and other mycobacterial species from ferrets and stoats. Vet Microbiol 2008;132:402–7.
33. Lucas J, Lucas A, Furber H, et al. *Mycobacterium genavense* infection in two aged ferrets with conjunctival lesions. Aust Vet J 2000;78:685–9.
34. Schultheiss PC, Dolginow SZ. Granulomatous enteritis caused by *Mycobacterium avium* in a ferret. J Am Vet Med Assoc 1994;204:1217–8.
35. Tappe JP, Weitzman I, Liu S, et al. Systemic *Mycobacterium marinum* infection in a European hedgehog. J Am Vet Med Assoc 1983;183:1280–1.
36. Heineman HS, Spitzer S, Pianphongsant T. Fish tank granuloma. A hobby hazard. Arch Intern Med 1972;130:121–3.
37. Jones JW, Pether JV, Rainey HA, et al. Recurrent *Mycobacterium bovis* infection following a ferret bite. J Infect 1993;26:225–6.

38. Salkelda DJ, Salathéb M, Stappc P, et al. Plague outbreaks in prairie dog populations explained by percolation thresholds of alternate host abundance. Can J Public Health 2001;92:67–71.
39. Williams ES, Mills K, Kwiatkowski DR, et al. Plague in a black-footed ferret (*Mustela nigripes*). J Wildl Dis 1994;30:581–5.
40. Duplantier JM, Duchemin JB, Chanteau S, et al. From the recent lessons of the Malagasy foci towards a global understanding of the factors involved in plague re-emergence. Vet Res 2005;36:437–53.
41. Keymer IF, Gibson EA, Reynolds DJ. Zoonoses and other findings in hedgehogs (*Erinaceus europaeus*): a survey of mortality and review of the literature. Vet Rec 1991;128:245–9.
42. Tertti R, Granfors K, Lehtonen OP, et al. An outbreak of *Yersinia pseudotuberculosis* infection. J Infect Dis 1984;149:245–50.
43. Tortem M. Leptospirosis. In: Steell JH, editor. CRC handbook series zoonosis. Cleveland: CRC Press; 1979.
44. Hathaway SC, Blackmore DK. Failure to demonstrate the maintenance of leptospires by free living carnivoos. N Z Vet J 1981;29:115–6.
45. Pepin GC, Austwick PKC. Skin diseases of domestic animals. II. Skin disease, mycological origin. Vet Rec 1968;82:208–14.
46. Silva-Hunter M, Weitzman I, Rosenthal SA. Cutaneous mycoses (dermatomycoses). In: Balows A, Hausler WJ Jr, editors. Diagnostic procedures for bacterial, mycotic and parasitic infections. 6th edition. Washington (DC): American Public Health Association; 1981.
47. Hagen KW, Gorham JR. Dermatomycosis in fur animals: chinchilla, ferret, mink and rabbit. Vet Med Small Anim Clin 1972;67:43–8.
48. Fox JG. Mycotic diseases. In: Fox JG, editor. Biology and diseases of the ferret. 2nd edition. Baltimore: Williams and Wilkins; 1998. p. 393–403.
49. Lewington JH. Viral, bacterial and mycotic diseases. In: Ferret husbandry, medicine and surgery. London: Butterworth; 1999. p. 105–28.
50. Besch-Williford CL. Biology and medicine of the ferret. In: Quesenberry KE, Hillyer EV, editors. Vet Clin North Am Small Anim Pract 1994;24:1155–83.
51. Kelleher SA. Skin diseases of ferrets. Vet Clin North Am Exot Anim Pract 2001;4: 565–72.
52. Lloyd M. Dermatologic diseases. In: Ferrets— health, husbandry and diseases. London: Blackwell Science; 1999. p. 78–87.
53. Marini RP, Adkins JA, Fox JG. Proven or potential zoonotic diseases of ferrets. J Am Vet Med Assoc 1989;195:990–4.
54. Orcutt C. Dermatologic diseases. In: Hillyer EV, Quesenberry KE, editors. Ferrets, rabbits and rodents— clinical medicine and surgery. Philadelphia: WB Saunders; 1997. p. 115–25.
55. Collins BR. Dermatologic disorders of common small non-domestic animals. In: Nesbitt GH, editor. Contemporary issues in small animal practice: dermatology. New York: Churchill Livingstone; 1987.
56. Rosen T. Hazardous hedgehogs. South Med J 2000;93:936–8.
57. Riley PY, Chomel BB. Hedgehog zoonoses. Emmerg Infect Dis 2005;11:1–5.
58. Lenhard A. Blastomycosis in a ferret. J Am Vet Med Assoc 1985;186:70–2.
59. Zoonoses and communicable diseases common to man and animals, vol. II: chlamydioses, rickettsioses, and viroses. 3rd edition. Washington (DC): Pan American Health Organization; 2001.
60. Doggart L. Viral disease of pet ferrets: part II. Aleutian disease, influenza, and rabies. Vet Technol 1988;8:384–9.

61. Marois P, Boudreault A, DiFranco E, et al. Response of ferrets and monkeys to intranasal infection with human, equine, and avian influenza viruses. Can J Comp Med 1971;35:71–6.
62. Shope RE. The infection of ferrets with swine influenza virus. J Exp Med 1934;60:49–61.
63. Zitzow LA, Rowe T, Morken T, et al. Pathogenesis of avian influenza A (H5N1) viruses in ferrets. J Virol 2002;76:4420–9.
64. Smith W, Andrews DH, Laidlow PO. The virus obtained from influenza patients. Lancet 1933;2:66.
65. Munster VJ, de Wit E, van den Brand JM, et al. Pathogenesis and transmission of swine-origin 2009 A(H1N1) influenza virus in ferrets. Science 2009;325:481–3.
66. Smith W, Stuart-Harris CH. Influenza infection of man from the ferret. Lancet 1936;2:21.
67. Smith H, Sweet C. Lessons for human influenza from pathogenicity studies in ferrets. Rev Infect Dis 1998;10:56–75.
68. Sweet C, Fenton RJ, Price GE. The ferret as an animal model of influenza virus infection. In: Zak O, Sande MA, editors. Handbook of animal models of infection. New York: Academic Press; 1999. p. 989–98.
69. Basarab O, Smith H. Quantitative studies on the tissue localization of influenza virus in ferrets after intranasal and intravenous or extracordial inoculation. Br J Exp Pathol 1969;50:612.
70. Marini RP, Adkins JA, Fox JG. Proven and potential zoonotic diseases of ferrets. J Am Vet Med Assoc 1989;195:990–4.
71. Collie MH, Rushton DI, Sweet C, et al. Studies of influenza infection in newborn ferrets. J Med Microbiol 1980;13:561–71.
72. Buchman CA, Swarts JD, Seroky JT, et al. Otologic and systemic manifestations of experimental influenza A virus infection in the ferret. Otolaryngol Head Neck Surg 1995;112:572–8.
73. Rosenthal KL. Respiratory disease. In: Quesenberry KE, Carpenter JW, editors. Ferrets, rabbits and rodents clinical medicine and surgery. 2nd edition. Philadelphia: WB Saunders; 2004. p. 72–8.
74. Sweet C, Macartney JC, Bird RA, et al. Differential distribution of virus and histological damage in the lower respiratory tract of ferrets infected with influenza viruses of differing virulence. J Gen Virol 1981;54:103–14.
75. Coates DM, Husseini RH, Rushton DI, et al. The role of lung development in the age related susceptibility of ferrets to influenza virus. Br J Exp Pathol 1984;65:543.
76. Sweet O, Jakeman KJ, Rushton I, et al. Role of upper respiratory tract infection in the deaths occurring in neonatal ferrets infected with influenza virus. Microb Pathog 1988;5:121–5.
77. Glathe H, Lebhardt A, Hilgenfeld M, et al. Intestinal influenza infection in ferrets (in German). Arch Exp Veterinar Med 1984;38:771–7.
78. Sweet C, Bird RA, Cavanah D, et al. The local origin of the febrile response induced in ferrets during respiratory infection with a virulent influenza virus. Br J Exp Pathol 1979;60:300.
79. Husseini RH, Sweet C, Overton H, et al. Role of maternal immunity in the protection of newborn ferrets against infection with a virulent influenza virus. Immunology 1984;52:389–94.
80. Hulse EC, Edwards JT. Foot-and-mouth disease in hibernating hedgehogs. J Comp Pathol 1937;50:421–30.
81. McLauchlan JD, Henderson WM. The occurrence of foot-and-mouth disease in the hedgehog under natural conditions. J Hyg (Lond) 1947;45:474–9.
82. Elgart ML. Scabies. Dermatol Clin 1990;8:253–63.

83. Zoonoses and communicable diseases common to man and animals, vol. III: Arasitoses, Third Edition. Washington (DC): Pan American Health Organization.
84. Oglesbee BL. The 5-minute veterinary consult: ferret and rabbit. Ames (IA): Blackwell Publishing; 2006.
85. Patterson M, Fox JG. Parasites of ferrets. In: Baker DG, editor. Flynn's parasites of laboratory animals. 2nd edition. Ames (IA): Blackwell Publishing; 2007.
86. Marini RP, Otto G, Erdman S, et al. Biology and diseases of ferrets. In: Fox JG, Anderson LC, Loew FM, et al, editors. Laboratory animal medicine. 2nd edition. Amsterdam: Academic Press; 2002. p. 483–517.
87. Orcutt C. Dermatologic diseases. In: Carpenter JW, Quesenberry KE, editors. Ferrets, rabbits, and rodents: clinical medicine and surgery. 2nd edition. St. Louis: Saunders; 2000. p. 107–14.
88. Hoppmann E, Barron HW. Ferret and rabbit dermatology. J Exotic Pet Med 2007; 16:225–37.
89. Paterson S. Skin diseases of exotic pets. Ames (IA): Blackwell Science; 2006. p. 204–9.
90. Bexton S, Robinson I. Hedgehogs. In: BSAVA Manual of Wildlife Casualties. Mullimeux: British Small Animal Veterinary Association; 2003.
91. Ellis C, Mori M. Skin diseases of rodents and small exotic mammals. Vet Clin North Am Exot Anim Pract 2001;4:523–7.
92. Isenbugel E, Baumgartner RA. Diseases of the hedgehog. In: Fowler ME, editor. Zoo and wild animal medicine: current therapy. Philadelphia: W. B. Saunders Company; 1993. p. 284–302.
93. Johnson-Delaney CA. Other small mammals. In: Meredith A, Redrobe S, editors. BSAVA manual of exotic pets. Gloucester: British Small Animal Veterinary Association; 2002. p. 108–12.
94. Barriga OO. Veterinary parasitology for practitioners, 2nd edition. Edina (MN): Burgess International Group; 1997.
95. Benenson AS, editor. Control of communicable diseases manual. 16th edition. An official report of the American Public Health Association. Washington, DC: American Public Health Association; 1995.
96. Clavel A, Arnal AC, Sanchez EC, et al. Respiratory cryptosporidiosis: case series and review of the literature. Infection 1996;24:341–6.
97. Abe N, Iseki M. Identification of genotypes of *Cryptosporidium parvum* isolates from ferrets in Japan. Parasitol Res 2003;89:422–4.
98. Graczyk TK, Cranfield MR, Dunning C, et al. Fatal cryptosporidiosis in a juvenile captive African hedgehog (*Ateletrix albiventris*). J Parasitol 1998;84:178–80.
99. Hoefer HL, Bell JA. Gastrointestinal diseases. In: Carpenter JW, Quesenberry KE, editors. Ferrets, rabbits, and rodents: clinical medicine and surgery. 2nd edition. St. Louis: Saunders; 2000. p. 25–40.
100. Barriga OO. Veterinary parasitology for practitioners, 2nd edition. Edina (MN): Burgess International Group; 1997.
101. Flanagan PA. Giardia—diagnosis, clinical course and epidemiology. A review. Epidemiol Infect 1992;109:1–22.
102. Abe N, Read C, Thompson RCA, et al. Zoonotic genotype of *Giardia intestinalis* detected in a ferret. J Parasitol 2005;91:179–82.
103. Hill DR. Giardiasis: issues in diagnosis and management. Infect Dis Clin North Am 1993;7:503–25.
104. Johnson-Delaney CA. Practical marsupial medicine. Proceeding of the American Exotic Mammals Veterinarian Conference. Bonita Springs (FL); 2006. p. 51–60.
105. Meyer EA, Jarroll EL. Giardiasis. In: Jacobs L, Arámbulo P. CRC handbook series in zoonoses, vol. 1. Boca Raton (FL): CRC Press; 1982.

Zoonoses of Procyonids and Nondomestic Felids

Edward C. Ramsay, DVM, DACZM

- *Baylisascaris procyonis* • Nondomestic felid • Procyonid
- *Procyon lotor* • Raccoon • Zoonoses

Relatively few species in the Order Carnivora, other than domestic dogs, cats, and ferrets, are kept as pets, but members of the families Procyonidae and Felidae are the most likely nondomestic carnivores to be kept by private owners. Additionally, many nondomestic felids and procyonids are exhibited by zoos and native wildlife parks. In the wild, contact with nondomestic felids is rare, but wild raccoons are common throughout North America and frequently found near human dwellings and parks. Reports of zoonoses transmitted from procyonids and nondomestic felids are uncommon, with a few notable exceptions. As with any zoonosis, immunocompromised individuals and children are at the greatest risk of acquiring zoonoses, and particular effort must be made to avoid infections in these people.

PROCYONIDS

The family Procyonidae contains small- to medium-sized omnivores that live in the temperate and tropical regions of the Western Hemisphere. The best-known member of this group is the common raccoon, *Procyon lotor*, which lives throughout North America and has feral populations established in Japan and Europe. Other species of procyonids live in the West Indies, and Central and South America. The coat mundi, *Nasua nasua*, is similar in size to the raccoon and ranges from Arizona to Argentina. The kinkajou, *Potto flavus*, and the olingos, *Bassaricyon* spp, are smaller, mostly arboreal procyonids of Central and South America. This family also includes the rarely seen ring-tailed cats, *Bassariscus* spp, from western North and Central America.

Raccoons are the most common privately owned procyonid seen in our practice and are popular exhibit animals worldwide. Wild raccoons live in urban, suburban, and rural areas and are well adapted to living in close proximity to people. Raccoons will feed on garbage and also use bird feeders and unattended pet food as food sources. Increased interactions with raccoons are likely as human populations continue to expand. It is estimated that the raccoon population of the United States will double over the next 10 years.[1] Kinkajous are prehensile-tailed procyonids and

Vet Clin Exot Anim 14 (2011) 551-556
doi:10.1016/j.cvex.2011.05.002
1094-9194/11/$ – see front matter © 2011 Elsevier Inc. All rights reserved.

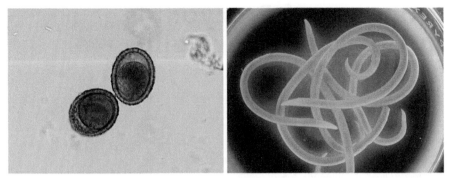

Fig. 1. Ova (left) and adult *Baylisascaris procyonis* from a raccoon. (*Courtesy of* The University of Tennessee, College of Veterinary Medicine's Parasitology Laboratory, Knoxville, TN.)

occasionally kept as pets. Other procyonids are rarely kept in the United States but may be kept as pets within their range countries. The discussion of zoonoses in this section will refer almost strictly to raccoons, alluding to kinkajous where data is available.

Raccoons are susceptible to most zoonotic diseases that infect domestic dogs. Serological surveys have also identified wild raccoons infected with a number of less common zoonotic agents, including *Bartonella rochalimaea*,[2] *Francisella tularensis*,[3] influenza virus,[4] *Trichinella spiralis*,[5] and *Trypanosoma cruzi*.[6] Of these minor zoonotic pathogens, *Ehrlichia chaffeensis* is probably the only organism for which raccoons are a potential reservoir host.[7]

Remarkably, there are very few reports of humans acquiring infections from raccoons, with the exceptions of 2 pathogens: rabies and the ascarid, *B procyonis*. Rabies is endemic in raccoons in the eastern portion of the United States and is discussed in another chapter in this book.

B procyonis

B procyonis is an enteric nematode parasite of raccoons (**Fig. 1**) and has recently been found in a pet kinkajou (Marcy Souza, personal communication, 2011). Domestic dogs have also been found to shed *B procyonis* ova.[8] *B procyonis* ova are very hardy and can remain infective in the environment for a long time; making exposure possible long after raccoons are gone. Reported infection prevalence rates in raccoons range up to 85%, with the western, upper Midwest and northeastern parts of the United States having the greatest reported prevalences.[9] *B procyonis* can have a direct life cycle, but raccoons are most likely to acquire this organism via ingestion of an intermediate host such as an infected rodent. Raccoon infections are typically asymptomatic but younger animals have heavier parasite infections and may show clinical signs. Infected raccoons may pass thousands of *B procyonis* ova.[10] Diagnosis of infection in procyonids is by identification of characteristic ova on fecal flotation exam or by direct observation of the adult worms at necropsy.

People acquire *B procyonis* by ingestion of infective ova. Individuals with a propensity to eating dirt or soil (geophagia), such as very young children or mentally handicapped individuals, are at greatest risk for infection. Most human infections appear to be asymptomatic.[11] Severe clinical presentations are the result of visceral, ocular, or neural larval migrans. Visceral larval migration may affect the heart, lungs, intestines, or mesenteries. Ocular larval migration may cause choroidoretinitis or optic neuritis and may result in visual defects or even blindness.[12,13] Fewer than 20 cases of neural larval migrans have been reported in North America, but most of those cases have resulted in death or persistent, severe neurological deficits. All reports of neural larval migrans have been in males, and either were children or mentally challenged individuals. Treatment of exposed individuals before the onset of clinical signs with albendazole may be useful.[10]

There are several strategies for preventing human infection with *B procyonis*. Avoiding raccoon latrines and contact with raccoon feces or contaminated areas are the most straight forward methods to avoid infection. Young children and others at increased risk of ingesting ova should be supervised when outside in areas with high raccoon activity. People should not intentionally feed wild raccoons and should avoid practices that attract raccoons, such as leaving human and pet food outdoors overnight. Garbage containers should have tight lids and remain sealed overnight. Sealing off or raccoon proofing areas, such as garages and unattended barns, may prevent the development of raccoon latrines near homes. Removal of raccoon latrines and treatment of potential intermediate rodent hosts is another strategy for reducing the risk of infection in people.[14]

NONDOMESTIC FELIDS

The family Felidae contains approximately 3 dozen species, which are native to all continents except Australia. The genus *Panthera* contains the charismatic large cats: lions (*Panthera leo*), tigers (*Panthera tigris*), leopards (*Panthera pardus* and *Panthera uncia*), and jaguars (*Panthera onca*). The cheetah (*Acinonyx jubatus*) is a distinctive felid and the only member of its genus. The taxonomy of the remainder of the felids is under seemingly continuous debate, but some have included all these smaller cats in a single genus, *Felis*. All felids are strict carnivores.

Nondomestic felids are not recommended as pets, but several species can be legally acquired and are occasionally kept by private individuals. Two small, attractive American felids, the ocelot (*Felis pardalis*) and margay (*Felis wiedii*), were once popular but are now seldom seen as pets. Servals (*Felis serval*), caracals (*Felis caracal*), and mountain lions (also known as the cougars or puma, *Felis concolor*) are the most commonly seen privately owned nondomestic felids in our practice.

All nondomestic felids appear to be susceptible to diseases commonly infecting domestic cats. As such, any zoonosis that might be acquired from domestic cats could potentially be acquired from nondomestic felids. Very few zoonoses, however, have been documented as contracted from a nondomestic felid. Two groups of pathogens, dermatophytes and enteric organisms, deserve mention as risks when working with exotic felids. Of the latter, knowledge of the biology of *Toxoplasma gondii* is frequently required for counseling owners of exotic felids and animal keepers.

DERMATOPHYTOSIS

Microsporum canis is a keratophilic fungus that causes superficial skin infections in domestic cats and dogs and has been the dermatophyte most commonly associated with disease in exotic felids. Dermatophytosis in exotic cats is similar to the disease in domestic cats, and lesions can include papular and miliary dermatitis or areas of alopecia on the face, body, and limbs.[15] Inapparent carriers may also exist. Diagnosis is made by clinical signs and fungal culture of lesions.

In most cases, infections appear to be self-limiting. Treatment may be attempted for severe or complicated cases; however, in one study of topical treatments of tigers and their outdoor exhibits, untreated (control group) animals resolved infections as fast as

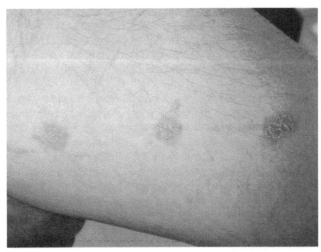

Fig. 2. The arm of a veterinarian infected with *Microsporum canis*, acquired from a tiger (*Panthera tigris*).

or faster than any treated tigers.[15] Focal lesions on kittens can be clipped, cleaned with a tamed iodine solution such as povidone iodine, and treated with topical antifungal agents such as miconazole or clotrimazole. Systemic treatment with oral itraconazole will speed resolution of lesions in adult cats. Griseofulvin toxicity causing bone marrow depression and death has been reported in cheetahs.[16]

Dermatophytosis in people is characterized as focal, circular skin lesions (**Fig. 2**), but lesions may also include alopecia. Inflammation may be minimal to intense, with vesicles and/or scaling present. The lesions can be pruritic. Diagnosis is based on history of exposure to infected animals, clinical signs, and fungal cultures. Physicians should be consulted regarding treatment. Wearing protective clothing and gloves and otherwise avoiding direct contact with infected cats is advised. Frequent handwashing following contact with infected felids also appears to limit zoonotic infections.

ENTERIC PATHOGENS

Toxocara cati and hookworms, *Ancylostoma* spp, are common zoonotic parasites of domestic cats and have been found in several species of nondomestic felids.[17] *T cati* infections rarely cause clinical signs in exotic felids but can be persistent, despite aggressive anthelminthic treatment. Infectious ascarid ova can be sequestered in an exhibit's crevices or substrate and remain infective for months to years, even in the most diligently cleaned enclosures.

T cati and hookworms can cause visceral and cutaneous larval migrans, respectively, in people. Human infections with *T cati* are acquired through ingestion of infective ova. Hookworm infections most typically occur when free-living larvae penetrate the skin. Both infections are more common in individuals who might consume contaminated soil or have considerable exposure to contaminated earth, such as children. A number of common anthelminthics are used to treat human infections.

Nondomestic cats fed raw meat diets can commonly be asymptomatic carriers of *Salmonella* spp.[18] Diets are presumed to be the source of the bacteria, but cultures of food items do not always reveal the same organisms cultured from feces.

Salmonellosis may occur in felids, but more frequently they shed *Salmonella* spp without showing clinical signs. Providing diets with low bacterial contamination, such as by acquiring meat from processors with human food quality hygiene practices, will limit shedding of *Salmonella* spp in nondomestic felids.[19]

Gastrointestinal signs, such as vomiting and diarrhea, are the most common clinical presentations associated with salmonella infections in people. Systemic signs are seen in severe infections. No reports could be found of human salmonellosis acquired from an exotic felid.

Serologic surveys of our collections have shown nondomestic felids to be commonly infected with *Toxoplasma gondii*. Domestic cats are known to be the definitive host for this organism, and it is assumed that all felids may act as definitive hosts. Although no records of transmission of *T gondii* from exotic felids to humans could be found, veterinarians are frequently called upon to council private owners, animal caretakers, and zoological collection managers about the risks of people becoming infected, especially when owners or keepers are pregnant.

Cats recently infected with *T gondii* shed the organism in feces for 2 to 3 weeks. Oocysts require at least 24 hours outside the body to sporulate and become infective. Transmission to people occurs following consumption of infective oocysts. The vast majority of human toxoplasmosis infections cause few or only mild flulike signs and are not diagnosed. In immunocompromised individuals, severe clinical disease, including encephalitis, may occur. Infection during pregnancy may result in fetal infection and cause fetal death or miscarriage. In utero, toxoplasmosis can cause fetal chorioretinitis and result in blindness of the neonate.

Avoiding contact with cat feces is the primary method to avoid infection with all enteric pathogens. Frequent hand washing and not eating, drinking, or smoking while feeding felids or cleaning enclosures will limit an individual's exposure to these agents. Wearing gloves when both cleaning cat boxes or enclosures and digging in soils contaminated with cat feces is also recommended. Hookworm infections can be avoided by wearing shoes in areas contaminated with cat feces. Animal keepers feeding felids raw meat should wear gloves when handling diets.

BITES

As with any wild animal, care must be taken when dealing with procyonids and nondomestic felids to avoid injury to the owner, technicians, and the veterinarian. Heavy leather gloves can be used to restrain smaller procyonids, but many can still bite through gloves. Even those animals most accustomed to captivity should be anesthetized or chemically restrained for physical examination and collection of biological samples. Procyonids and small felids can be netted and hand injected with anesthetic agents. Alternately, we frequently leave the animal in its transport container and place the entire container in a plastic bag, creating a type of anesthetic chamber. The bag is filled with inhalation anesthetic gases, such as isoflurane in oxygen, and the animal induced without needing to be handled. Larger felids typically require darting.

SUMMARY

There are very few reports of zoonotic diseases having been acquired from procyonids and nondomestic felids. *B procyonis* is the most commonly documented zoonotic agent in these taxa. Routine personal protective strategies, such as wearing gloves and avoiding contact with contaminated environments, remain the best strategies for preventing zoonotic infections from procyonids and nondomestic felids.

REFERENCES

1. Kenyon S, Southwick R, Wynne C. Bears in the backyard, deer in the driveway. International Assoc of Fish and Wildlife Agencies. Available at: http://georgiawildlife.org/node/2275. Accessed June 20, 2011.
2. Henn JB, Chomel BB, Boulouis H-J, et al. Bartonella rochalimae in raccoons, coyotes, and red foxes. Emerg Inf Dis 2009;15(12):1984-7.
3. Berrada ZL, Goethert HK, Telford SR III. Raccoons and skunks as sentinels for enzootic tularemia. Emerg Inf Dis 2006;12(6):1019-21.
4. Hall JS, Bentler KT, Landolt G, at al. Influenza infection in wild raccoons. Emerg Inf Dis 2008;14(12):1842-8.
5. Burke R, Masuoka P, Murrell KD. Swine Trichinella infection and geographic information system tools. Emer Inf Dis 2008;14(7):1109-11.
6. Yabsley MJ, Noblet GP. Biological and molecular characterization of a raccoon isolate of Trypanosoma cruzi from South Carolina. J Parasitol 2002;88(6):1273-6.
7. Kocan A, Levesque GC, Whitworth LC, et al. Naturally occurring Ehrlichia chaffeensis infection in coyotes from Oklahoma. Emerg Inf Dis 2000;6:477-80.
8. Greve JH, S O'Brien. Adult Baylisascaris infection in two dogs. Comp Anim Pract 1989;19:41-3.
9. Souza MJ, Ramsay EC, Patton S, et al. Baylisascaris procyonis in raccoons (Procyon lotor) in eastern Tennessee. J Wildl Dis 2010;45(4):1231-4.
10. Kazacos KR. Baylisascaris procyonis and related species. In: Samuel WM, Pybus MJ, Kocan AA, editors. Parasitic diseases of wild mammals. 2nd edition. Ames (IO), Iowa State University Press; 2001:301-41.
11. Brinkman WB, Kazacos KR, Gavin PJ, et al. Seroprevalence of Baylisascaris procyonis (raccoon roundworm) in Chicago area children. In: Program and Abstracts 2003 Ann Meeting Pediat Acad Soc. Seattle (WA), May 3-6, 2003 [abstract: 1872].
12. Goldberg, MA, KR Kazacos, WM Boyce, et al. Diffuse unilateral subacute neuritis. Morphometric, serologic and epidemiologic support for Baylisascaris as a causative agent. Ophthalmol 1993;100:1695-1701.
13. Mets MB, AG Noble, S Basti, et al. Eye findings of diffuse unilateral subacute neuroretinitis and multiple choroidal infiltrates associated with neural larva migrans due to Baylisascaris procyonis. Am J Ophthalmol 2003;135:888-90.
14. Page LK, Beasley JC, Olson ZH, et al. Reducing Baylisascaris procyonis roundworm larvae in raccoon latrines. Emerg Infect Dis 2011. Available at: http://www.cdc.gov/EID/content/17/90.htm. Accessed January 7, 2011.
15. Sykes JM, Ramsay EC. Attempted treatment of tigers (Panthera tigris) infected with Microsporum canis. J Zoo Wild Med 2007;38(2):252-7.
16. Wack R. Felidae. In: Fowler ME, Miller RE, editors. Current veterinary therapy in zoo and wildlife medicine. 5th edition. St Louis (MO): W.B. Saunders; 2005. p. 491501.
17. Greene CE, Levy JL. Immunocompromised people and shared human and animal infections: zoonoses, sapronoses, and anthroponoses. In: Greene CE, editor. Infectious diseases of the dog and cat. 3rd edition. St. Louis (MO): Elsevier, Inc; 1998. p. 1052-68.
18. Clyde VL, Ramsay EC, Bemis DA. Fecal shedding of Salmonella in exotic felids. J Zoo Wild Med 1997;28(2):148-52.
19. Lewis CE, Bemis DA, Ramsay EC. Positive effects of diet change on shedding of Salmonella spp in the feces of captive felids. J Zoo Wild Med 2007;38(2):252-7.

Zoonotic Diseases of Primates

Armando G. Burgos-Rodriguez, DVM ABVP-Avian

KEYWORDS
• Primates • Zoonoses • Viruses • Bacteria • Parasites
• Prevention

The World Health Organization defines a zoonotic disease as "any disease or infection that is naturally transmissible from vertebrate animals to humans; animals thus play an essential role in maintaining zoonotic infections in nature."[1] According to the literature, of the identified 1407 human pathogens, 58% are zoonotic.[2] Both of these statements show the significance of zoonotic diseases to both veterinary and human medicine, and the public health.

This article focuses on pertinent zoonotic diseases that have to be taken into consideration when working with nonhuman primate (NHP) species. Many factors may influence the occurrence of these diseases such as the origin of the species involved (Old World vs New World), location (zoologic park vs laboratory setting), and geography (Americas vs Africa). In addition, other factors such as international travel, loss of native habitat, importation of feral animals, and the immune status of both the animal and human may play a role in the prevalence of these diseases.

Primates are kept in captivity in zoologic parks, research facilities, and as pets. In addition, free-range or feral primate species in several countries have close human interaction. Zoonotic diseases of NHP origin can occur during occupational exposure, hunting, consumption of contaminated food, vector exposure, and leisure activities (ecotourism), among others.[3] Human and NHPs share many similarities, not only anatomically but also physiologically, which makes them both susceptible to many species-specific pathogens.[4–6] As a consequence, NHP are valuable models for many human infectious diseases; therefore, staff can be exposed to many potential pathogens.[6] Veterinary staff working with NHPs are exposed to zoonotic pathogens via bites, scratches, and accidental contact with body fluids (needle sticks, fluid exposure). In addition, some primates may carry latent viruses (B virus or Cercophith-ecine herpesvirus 1) that may pose serious health threats to personnel. In general, the disease state of a primate can range from asymptomatic carrier to death from infection.

Caribbean Primate Research Center, PO Box 1053, Sabana Seca, Puerto Rico 00952
E-mail address: armando.burgos@upr.edu

Vet Clin Exot Anim 14 (2011) 557-575
doi:10.1016/j.cvex.2011.05.006
1094-9194/11/$ – see front matter © 2011 Elsevier Inc. All rights reserved.

POTENTIAL IMPACT OF ZOONOTIC DISEASES

NHPs can serve as a potential reservoir of zoonotic diseases and approximately 25% of the human emerging infectious diseases are shared with primate host species.[7] Zoonotic diseases are not only a concern to an individual, but also to the general population. Some of these diseases may serve as potential bioterrorism agents, which in some cases have high morbidity and mortality. Viral or bacterial infections pose a risk of exposure to large populations from inhalation or contaminated foodstuffs.[6]

Emergence of zoonotic diseases is an important aspect of concern for both veterinary and human medicine and is influenced by several factors. Host–pathogen interaction plays a key role in the establishment of such infections. Naive hosts may lack an appropriate immune response, resulting in a rapid spread of the disease and high virulence.[7] Anytime that there is close human–animal interactions, a risk of cross-species infection is present. Several viruses such as simian immunodeficiency virus (SIV), simian T-lymphotrophic virus (STLV)-1 and Ebola serve as examples.[7] The immune status of the animal plays an important role in the occurrence of zoonotic diseases. Many etiologies that lead to immunodeficiency may result in bacteremias and sepsis.[8] An additional factor that may influence the emergence of zoonotic disease, particularly those of bacterial origin, is resistance to antibiotics.[9]

Xenotransplantation, although not a common route of zoonotic disease infection, needs to be considered as well. In terms of risks, viruses present the largest risk of spread of zoonotic diseases in transplants.[10] Retroviruses currently cannot be removed from the donor tissue and these viruses may affect a potential recipient.

BACTERIAL AGENTS
Mycobacterium spp

One of the most significant zoonotic diseases in primate medicine is tuberculosis. It is important not only because of its impact on a primate colony but also humans working around infected animals. Tuberculosis is one of the diseases with both zoonotic and anthropozoonotic (a disease spread from humans to animals) potential.[11] According to the US Centers for Disease Control and Prevention, each year over 9 million people become infected with tuberculosis and almost 2 million die worldwide.[12] Tuberculosis is caused by a gram positive acid-fast bacillus of the Mycobacterium species, with M tuberculosis being the most common isolate reported in NHP.[4,5,11,13] Other isolates such as M bovis have also been reported in primates.[13] Old World primates seem more susceptible than New World primates to Mycobacterium, although infection in New World primates has been reported.[4,5,11,14] Aerosol transmission through the respiratory tract is the most common, although other routes of exposure such as ingestion and contact with infected fluid or tissues are also possible.[4,5,11,13,14] In zoologic settings, infection in several species can be devastating to a collection. In 1 report, many different species, including elephants, reptiles, and NHPs, were all affected in the same facility.[11] In that epizootic, 4 human infections occurred, with one of the veterinarians developing the disease after performing a necropsy on an infected monkey.

Tuberculosis can be present in an active or latent form. In active disease, clinical signs are more often associated with the respiratory tract (cough, dyspnea), but can also involve the gastrointestinal tract (weight loss). In the latent phase of the disease, no clinical signs are evident unless the immune system is affected.[12] Diagnosis of tuberculosis can be difficult; the intradermal skin test is currently the standard for testing animals, although false-negative results can occur.[4,5,14] A rhesus macaque

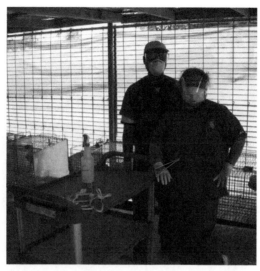

Fig. 1. Basic personal protection equipment is essential when working with NHPs.

that had 17 negative tuberculin tests was later euthanized for signs of pneumonia.[13] Several granulomas were present in the lung, liver, and spleen with a positive culture for *M bovis*. Animals housed in the same enclosure converted from a negative to positive tuberculin test. False-negative results with the intradermal test can occur with overwhelming infection owing to immunosupression.[4,5,15] False-positive tests can result from traumatic administration of the intradermal test, atypical mycobacteriosis infection, or the use of adjuvant-containing mycobacterial products (Andres Mejia DVM, MS, DACLAM, Toa Baja, PR, personal communication, January 2011). Additional commercial tests such as the PRIMAGAM (Prionics AG, Zurich, Switzerland) and PrimaTB STAT-PAK (Chembio Diagnostic Systems, Medford, NY, USA) are also available, but are not replacements for the intradermal skin test.[14] Quarantine of newly arrived animals is an important preventive measure, as well as full necropsies of suspect animals. Personnel working with NHPs should have a tuberculin skin test twice a year. Positive or suspect individuals should be further evaluated with chest radiographs and sputum cultures at a public or occupational health clinic and treatment instituted if positive results are obtained. These individuals should not be allowed to work with NHPs until cleared of infection. Personal protection equipment such as masks, gloves, and eye protection should be worn at all times when working with NHP **(Fig. 1)**.

Clostridium tetani

Tetanus is caused by an anaerobic, gram-positive, spore-forming bacillus that produces an exotoxin responsible for the disease.[16] The organism is shed in the feces of NHP, humans, and many other species, and can remain viable in spore form in the soil for many years.[4,5,16] NHP housed outdoors are at a higher risk[16,17] **(Fig. 2)**. Penetrating skin wounds (bites, scratches) can lead to infection, and infected tissue provides an adequate environment for toxin production. Neurologic signs often develop and may lead to respiratory compromise. In a free-range rhesus macaque colony with high incidence of *C tetani* infection, mass immunization proved to be

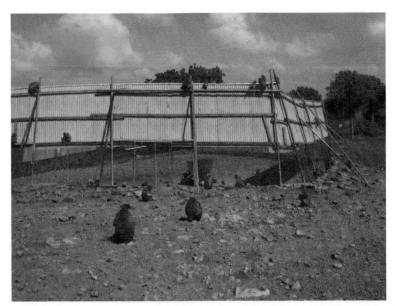

Fig. 2. Primates housed outdoors are at a higher risk of exposure to *C tetani*; this particular colony mass immunization proved to be effective in reducing significantly clinical cases of tetanus.

effective in eliminating clinical cases and drastically reducing the mortality rate.[17] Personnel working with NHP should be vaccinated against tetanus because of the inherent risk[18]; a diphtheria–tetanus toxoid at 10-year intervals can reduce the risk of toxin exposure. In addition, wounds that may occur while working with NHP (animal bite or scratch, cage scratch, needle puncture) or that may come in contact with soil or feces should be thoroughly rinsed and evaluated by a physician.

ENTERIC PATHOGENS

In NHP, one of the leading causes of morbidity and mortality is diarrhea. This condition can be caused by many enteric pathogens such as *Shigella*, *Salmonella*, *Escherichia coli*, and *Campylobacter* among others.[4,5,19,20] In a retrospective study of rhesus macaques, a high incidence of *Campylobacter spp*, *Shigella flexneri*, and *Yersinia enterocolitica* was present in animals with diarrhea.[20] Asymptomatic carriers of enteric pathogens also occur, and these carriers may develop diarrhea during periods of stress.[14,20,21] These organisms can cause enterocolitis in both NHP and humans with transmission via the fecal–oral route and is a concern because of its zoonotic potential, as well as its anthropozoonotic risk.[4,5,20–22] Personnel with diarrhea should not be allowed to work with NHP until symptoms have resolved. In severe cases, a fecal culture may be required to rule out any potential pathogen that may affect the colony or collection. To minimize the risk of infection with such pathogens, personnel should always wear gloves, eye protection, and masks. After working with any NHP, it is important to thoroughly wash hands or any contact surface as a preventive measure. The role of vermin as a source of spread of the bacteria cannot be underestimated, particularly in outdoor enclosures.

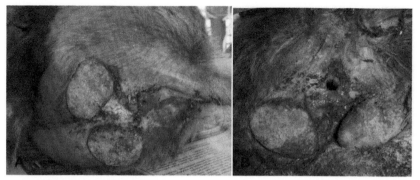

Fig. 3. (A) Evidence of mild rectal prolapse in a rhesus macaque with *Shigellosis*. (B) Rhesus monkey with hematochezia and mucus.

Shigella spp

Shigellosis is caused by a gram-negative, non–spore-forming bacilli.[4,5,23] In NHP, *S flexneri* is the most common isolate recovered from feces, but other species such as *S dysenteriae*, *S boydii*, and *S sonnei* have also been isolated.[4,5,21,22] Shigellosis is a highly communicable disease, in part because of its small inoculum size.[24] In humans, as few as 10 to 10^2 organisms have been implicated with infection. Clinical signs present both in NHP and humans include hematochezia with mucus, abdominal pain, and weight loss[19,23,25] (**Fig. 3**). In rhesus macaques, abortion, gingivitis, and air sac infection are also other forms of the disease.[15] In some scenarios, the presence of *Shigella* organisms in a collection may be enzootic in nature, which may cause epizootics in times of stress.[19] A similar situation occurs in humans living in developing countries leading to infection, particularly among children under 5 years of age.[25] Shigellosis has been reported in laboratory personnel working with NHP where fecally contaminated aerosol was suggested as the route of tranmission.[23] Treatment often includes fluid administration and antibiotics. A concern with *Shigella* organisms is the level of resistance present in some strains.[26]

Salmonellosis

Salmonellosis is caused by a gram-negative rod that can be found in feces, but also can be present in blood and urine.[4,5] The bacteria has the ability to survive and multiply in moist organic material.[4,5] Most cases are treated symptomatically, and, as with *Shigella* infections, antibiotic resistance is a concern in treatment options.[21] Asymptomatic carriers of the bacteria are also common.[22]

Escherichia coli

E coli is a gram-negative rod that can be present in the normal flora of NHP.[15] Clinical signs seen in apes include mucosal hemorrhage in the gastrointestinal tract, congested and enlarged mesenteric lymph nodes, and pulmonary hemorrhage and edema.[15] There are different strains of *E coli* that are classified according to the lesions they produce. These strains include enteropathogenic *E coli*, enterohemorrhagic *E coli*, enteroaggregative *E coli*, enterotoxigenic *E coli*, enteroinvasive *E coli*, Shiga-toxin–producing *E coli*, and diffusely adhering *E coli*.[14] Enteropathogenic *E coli* can be overlooked during routine culture if lactose-fermenting organisms are not speciated from fecal samples.[14] Some serotypes of *E coli* have been associated with severe human

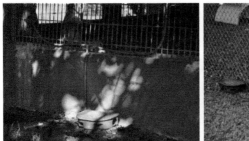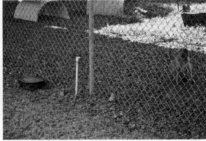

Fig. 4. Rodents traps need to placed in areas where no primates can have access to them.

illnesses, such as bloody diarrhea and hemolytic uremic syndrome, although these cases are mostly associated with cattle and are foodborne in origin.[27,28]

Campylobacter spp

Campylobacter is a small, gram-negative, non–spore-forming, spirally curved rod; *C jejuni* is most common isolate from NHP.[4,5] *C jejuni* and *C coli* have been isolated from clinical and subclinical NHP.[15] Infections in NHP can be self-limiting but reinfection can occur. *Campylobacter* is capable of growing at 43°C and has been shown to cause human enteritis, particularly in children and immunosuppressed adults.[4,5,21] Although infection can occur in personnel working with NHP, most of the human infections are from ingestion of undercooked poultry or cross-contamination with such food items.[29]

Other Bacteria

Yersinia enterocolitica is a gram-negative, unencapsulated, ovoid- to rod-shaped bacteria and is difficult to isolate in fecal culture. The bacteria can be found in both clinically healthy and sick animals.[4,5] Humans and NHP share the same pathogenic respiratory bacteria such as *Streptococcus pneumonia*, *Bordetella bronchioseprica*, *Pasteurella multocida*, *Staphylococcus aureus*, *Klebsiella pneumonia*, and *Hemophilus influenza*, making both zoonotic and anthropozoonotic infections a possibility.[4,5]

Leptospirosis, although uncommon in NHP, has been reported in several species of Old and New World primates. [30–32] The infection rate of New World primates is thought to be lower because of their arboreal nature.[32] In addition, experimental infection has shown that some species of NHP may be resistant to the infection or have only mild clinical signs, whereas others such as the squirrel monkey (*Saimiri sciureus*), are highly susceptible to disease.[31] In a breeding colony of squirrel monkeys, necropsy findings of affected animals included pneumonia, renal hemorrhage, jaundice, diffuse hemorrhage, and hepatomegaly. Antibodies were also found in 2 females that had miscarriages.[31] Rodents are the most common source of leptospiras, although other animals can also be carriers; vermin control is important for prevention of spread of the organism in a facility. The author has worked with an outdoor colony of rhesus macaques and has not seen any confirmed cases of leptospirosis despite the presence of rodents. A small survey from a group of rhesus macaques at the Caribbean Primate Research Center has shown positive serology for *Leptospira* organism, but no clinical cases. Rodent control is present around the premises, but complete rodent elimination is not possible owing to the nature and environment of the facility (**Fig. 4**). Possible causes for lack of clinical cases may be natural immunity in the colony, species resistance, or a low prevalence of *Leptospira* infection in the rodents.

Tularemia is caused by the infectious agent *Francisella tularensis*, which is transmitted via inoculation, ingestion, or inhalation.[33,34] Although not a common disease in NHP, it has been reported in several species and it has zoonotic potential.[33,35] In a report where several animals were affected with *F tularensis*, the attending veterinarian contracted the disease after being bitten by a tamarin.[35] Infection can be established in rodents, rabbits, blood-sucking arthropods, and contaminated water, making animals kept in outdoor enclosures susceptible to the disease. In an epizootic of tularemia in cynomolgus monkeys (*Macaca fascicularis*), pathologic findings resembled human infection and included ulceroglandular syndrome with local lymphade-nopathy, gingivostomatitis, and systemic spread, with manifestations such as subacute necrotizing hepatitis, granulomatous splenitis, and pneumonia.[33] Vector and vermin control are important to avoid introduction of such bacteria.

VIRAL AGENTS

Because of the close relation between humans and NHP, there is a potential for infection with any virus of NHP origin.[4,5] In addition, RNA viruses have a higher nucleotide substitution rate, which permits a more rapid adaptation, thus increasing the probability of invading a new host.[2] Research has shown that several human viruses such as HIV and HTLV have close links to their simian counterpart.[3]

Viral Anthropozoonotic Potential

Viruses, as well as some bacteria, have anthropozoonotic potential (the ability to be transmitted from human to animal), which plays an important role in the education of veterinary staff, employees, clients, and visitors. Such viruses with anthropozoonotic potential include measles, herpes, and other paramyxoviruses.[4,5,36–38]

Of greatest significance is measles because its devastating effects on a NHP colony. Clinical signs seen in Old World primates include conjunctivitis, maculopap-ular rash, white eruptions in the oral cavity (Koplik spots), diarrhea, and pneumo-nia.[13,36,39] Immunosuppression is another potential sequelae of measles infection leading to secondary bacterial and fungal infections. In New World primates, clinical signs may not be as obvious, and disease is often due to secondary infections after immunosupression.[13,39] Although human vaccination has drastically reduced the risk for infection, it should still be kept as a potential differential diagnosis in cases with the descr bed clinical presentation. Measles is transmitted via inhalation of respiratory droplets, nasal secretions, and contact with contaminated surfaces.[36] Because children are the demographic group most likely to be infected with measles, caution should be taken with children visiting NHP exhibits in zoologic parks. Although mass vaccination helped in an outbreak of measles in Old World primates, routine measles vaccination remains controversial.[38] Of the different primate centers around the United States and Caribbean, vaccination for measles is inconsistent, with some centers vaccinating and others not. As mentioned, vaccination in people remains the best preventive measure to avoid infection with the virus.

Two additional paramyxoviruses have been shown to infect NHP.[37] Human respiratory syncytial virus and human metapneumovirus were detected in wild chimpanzees that died during a respiratory disease outbreak in Côte d'Ivoire from 1999 to 2006.

Although herpesvirus in NHP infection is usually associated with the zoonotic potential of B virus, anthropozoonotic herpes virus infection can occur.[40] A 2-year-old male marmoset (*Callithrix jacchus*) died after developing severe necrotizing stomatitis, vomiting, and loss

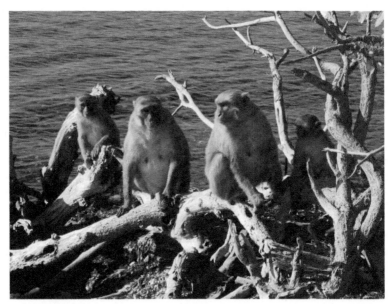

Fig. 5. *Cercopithecine herpesvirus* 1, or B virus, is enzootic in rhesus macaques (*Macaca mulatta*) and rarely causes clinical disease in these species.

of appetite several days after biting the owner. Virus isolation revealed human herpesvirus 1. Similar cases have also been reported in other marmosets.

Viral Zoonotic Potential

Herpesvirus

As illustrated, this class of virus has the ability to have asymptomatic carriers in 1 species of primates and cause fatal disease in another.[4,5,40] The most significant zoonotic viral disease in NHP, particularly in Old World primates, is *Cercopithecine herpesvirus* 1, or B virus, owing to its potential to cause fatal disease. Although the majority of macaques are used in research facilities and limited human exposure occurs, free-range or feral populations and exotic animals in the pet trade may expose the general population to this virus. The herpes B virus can be enzootic in primates of the genus *Macaca* and rarely produces diseases in these species[6,41] (**Fig. 5**). Infection in wild and captive macaques increases with age and is usually acquired by sexual maturity, at approximately 2 to 4 years of age. Oral lesions such as gingivostomatitis, oral or lingual ulcers, and conjunctivitis can be present in macaques but usually are associated with immunosuppression or stress (recent importation).[41] Although the incidence of human infection is low, its death rate makes herpes B virus a true concern. Human infection can result in fatal encephalomyelitis leading to respiratory failure associated with ascending paralysis.[41] Clinical symptoms can include influenza-like symptoms, fever, muscle aches, headache, nausea, vomiting, and abdominal pain.[4,5,41] Transmission is usually from bite wounds or scratches from infected animals,[4,5] but indirect contact (ie, needle puncture, cage scratch, mucosal contact) has also caused infection.[41]

Of particular interest is the fact that there have been no reported cases of herpes B virus in travelers to countries with frequent human–NHP interaction, even though

NHP bites do occur.[42] In a study by the GeoSentinel Surveillance Network, the second most frequently involved species in animal-related injuries to humans were monkeys.[42] This emphasizes the need for caution when traveling to places where primates may be free roaming. Despite frequent reports of injuries from NHP, herpes B virus infection has not been reported and arguments to explain this include: A less virulent B virus, minimal shed of virus by a wild NHP, or underdiagnosed cases of encephalitis. Similarly, exposure by a group of people to a herpes B virus confirmed feral rhesus macaque in Puerto Rico yielded no positive cases of herpes B virus in humans; however, most of the exposures were via blood and B virus is not a known blood pathogen.[43] If B virus exposure is suspected, medical personnel need to be familiar with this virus to avoid delayed use of antiviral medications. Also, inexperienced medical personnel may confuse B virus with hepatitis B instead of herpes B if it is only referred as "B virus." In cases of possible human exposure, cleansing the wound immediately and thoroughly flushing with iodine or chlorhexidine for 15 minutes must be performed to avoid entrance of the virus into the wound. If ocular splash occurs, rinsing with eye wash for the same amount of time is recommended.

Filoviruses
Marburg and Ebola are the most significant viruses in this group. Although not a common zoonotic agent, the potentially devastating effects of filoviruses makes them worth mentioning. According to the literature, 23 outbreaks of both viruses have been reported involving humans and NHP since 1967.[44] Most of the outbreaks occurred where contact with wild primate populations was more common, although outbreaks associated with contact with NHP used for scientific purposes have occurred.

The exact reservoir for these filoviruses remains currently unknown, although fruitbats have been theorized as potential reservoir in Ebola.[42] Common clinical presentation in both human and NHP include hemorrhagic syndrome (high fever, epistaxis, ecchymoses, gastrointestinal tract bleeding).[4,5] Marburg virus has been detected in blood, saliva, urine, and feces and experimentally is fatal to several species of primates. A closely related virus to Ebola was detected in a cynomolgus macaque (*Macaca fascicularis*) imported from the Philippines. This animal was held in a quarantine facility in Virginia and Pennsylvania. Several NHP died; no human deaths occurred, but serologic evidence of a recent filovirus infection was present.[4,5]

Yellow fever
Yellow fever is a flavivirus present in tropical areas (Americas and Africa) and is transmitted by the mosquito of *aedes Spp*. Most NHPs are susceptible to the infection and may serve as resorvoirs.[4,5] Clinical signs in both NHP and humans include fever, vomiting, yellow to green urine, albuminuria, and jaundice.[4,5,45] In humans, the disease has a high mortality rate, and between 1990 and 1999, 1939 cases and 941 deaths were reported in Peru.[43] A recent epizootic in both human and howler monkeys in Venezuela was caused by this virus.[46] Caution should be taken with animals imported from locations known to be endemic for the virus.

Hepatitis virus
Five different human hepatitis (A, B, C, D, and E) viruses have been described, all of which can be transmitted to Nhp.[4] Although not all 5 have been reported as zoonotic agents, the risk of exposure in personnel working with NHP is a possibility. Infections are often associated with laboratory-related exposure (needle sticks, mucosal exposure, contact exposure of broken skin), although other routes of exposure such as

blood transfusion, ingestion (enteroviruses-hepatitis A and E) and contact with broken skin can occur.[4,5,47] Natural infection with hepatitis A has been reported in chimpanzees (Pan troglodytes), owl monkeys (Aotus trivirgatus), African green monkeys (Cercopithecus aethiops), cynomolgus (Macaca fascicularis), and rhesus (Macaca mulatta) macaques.[4,5] A human vaccine against hepatitis A is available and is often recommended for at-risk personnel working with NHP.[18] Hepatitis B virus infection has been reported in apes, chimpanzees, and humans, with asymptomatic carriers present in the NHP population.[4,5] Hepatitis B has been among the most frequent infections associated with laboratory personnel.[18] The virus has been detected in blood, saliva, semen, cerebrospinal fluid, and urine.[18] A vaccine is also available for hepatitis B and is recommended for personnel working with NHP.[48] Hepatitis E is a waterborne disease and is common in developing countries, although sporadic cases in the United States have occurred.[47,49] Experimental inoculation has led to hepatitis E infection in owl monkeys, cynomolgus macaques, and tamarins, showing the potential role of these animals as reservoirs.[5]

Callitrichid hepatitis

Callitrichid hepatitis, a virus of the family arenavirus, causes fatal disease in new world primates, particularly captive marmosets and tamarins.[50] According to the literature, 14 epizootics of the disease have occurred in 11 zoologic parks in North America. Infected animals developed hepatitis after coming in contact with mice infected with a variant of another arenavirus with zoonotic potential, lymphocytic choriomeningitis virus.[50] Seroconversion to this variant of lymphocytic choriomeningitis virus has occurred in caretakers involved in outbreaks of the disease. In addition, another report mentioned seroconversion of 2 veterinarians with exposure to the Callitrichid hepatitis virus; the humans had no evidence of overt disease.[4,5] The virus has been detected in blood, urine, feces, and cerebrospinal fluid of NHP.[4,5]

Retroviral Diseases

NHPs are known to be infected with several different types of retroviruses which have zoonotic potential.[51–54] Retroviruses are RNA viruses, and as previously, have the ability to replicate with a high nucleotide substitution rate, allowing rapid adaptation and increasing the probability of invading a new host. Human populations could be impacted by these newly adapted retroviruses, although no cases of such viruses has been reported. Retroviruses are divided into 2 subfamilies: The Orthoretroviridae, composed of 6 genera (Alpharetrovirus, Betaretrovirus, Gammaretrovirus, Deltaretrovirus, Epsilonretrovirus, and Lentivirus) and the Spumaretrovirinae, composed of the Spumauirus (foamy virus) genus.[53]

STLV

STLV is an oncovirus that has been reported in several species of wild and captive Old World primates with no reported natural cases in New World primates.[4,5,53] There are 3 groups of STLV—1, 2, and 3.[53] STLV-1 has been reported in Asian and African primates, and STLV-2 has only been reported in captive bonobos (Pan paniscus). STLV-3 has only been reported in some Old World species. There is a genetic relationship between STLV and its human counterpart HTLV.[54] It is believed that HTLV is a result of a cross-species infection from STLV; some references group both viruses as primate T-lymphotropic virus.[54] Potential routes of exposure that lead to cross-species infection includes: Contact with blood and fluids from infected animals during hunting, consumption of bushmeat, and keeping primates as pets.

Animals infected with STLV-1 developed persistent lymphocytosis, T-cell lymphomas, leukemia, lymphadenopathy, skin lesions, and splenomegaly.[53] In gorillas (Gorilla gorilla), a chronic wasting disease has been seen in STLV-1 cases.[53] Interspecies infection has been reported between macaques and baboons and resulted in an outbreak of malignant lymphoma in the baboons.[55] STLV-2 and -3 are currently not thought to be pathogenic to NHP. In human HTLV cases, type 1 causes T-cell leukemia and an associated myelopathy with a spastic paraperesis,[56] and HTLV-2 seems to be less pathogenic, although it does cause neurologic disease.[56] Establishing viral status of a primate collection assists in decreasing exposure or taking necessary precautions to avoid infection.

Simian retrovirus
Simian retrovirus (SRV) has 5 different serotypes (1–5) and has been reported in several species of NHP.[4,5] SRV has been associated with a chronic wasting syndrome together with immunodeficiency; opportunistic infections, necrotizing gingivitis with osteomyelitis, and retroperitoneal fibromatosis also resulted from the immundeficiency.[4,5,53] SRV has also been associated with cutaneous and retroperitoneal fibromatosis, necrotizing acute death, fever, anemia, neutropenia, lymphopenia, thrombocytopenia, hypoproteinemia, persistent diarrhea, lymphadenopathy, splenomegaly, weight loss, thymic atrophy, and fibroproliferative disorders in NHP. The virus is present in blood, urine, and fluids, and transmission can be via bite wounds, sexual contact, and trasplacentally.[4,5] Serologic evidence of SRV in personnel working with NHP has been shown, but no overt disease has been reported.[57] Similar to other retroviruses, establishing viral status of the animal is important for the health of a colony or collection and also because of its zoonotic potential.

SIV
SIV is a lentivirus that is related to HIV.[51] Different isolates of the virus exist partly owing to its ability to mutate.[4,5,51,53] SIV infection in the natural host typically causes lifelong, clinically inapparent infection, but when this virus crosses species, disease can occur.[6,53] Infection of SIV in sooty mangabeys (Cercocebus atys) caused no clinical disease but led to immunosuppression in macaques.[4,5] Peristent infection in 3 different NHP species caused disease only in one of these species, but when the virus was passed through another species (pig-tailed macaque), the resulting virus was virulent in all 3 species.[4,5] This ability to mutate could lead to devastating effects in both animal and human populations. Of particular interest is the role of SIV as a zoonotic agent leading to HIV infection in humans from cross-species infection. HIV types 1 and 2 originated zoonotically from cross-species transmission of SIV from infected chimpanzees (Pan troglodytes) and sooty mangabeys (Cercocebus atys) in Central and West Africa, respectively.[6,53]

According to the literature, 2 suspected cases of SIV infection in laboratory personnel have been reported.[51] Both employees had antibodies to the virus, with no evidence of clinical disease. One case was from an accidental needle stick while handling an SIV-infected monkey. In the second case, the employee had severe dermatitis and was being treated with corticosteroids; the employee handled SIV-infected blood products without gloves. This emphasizes the importance of personal protective equipment when working with NHP or biological products. Although New World primates do not seem to be natural hosts of the virus and they seem to be resistant to the virus based on in vitro studies, actual susceptibility to virus remains unknown.[58]

Spumavirus

Simian foamy viruses (SFV) are present in many NHP, including New World and Old World primates and prosimiams.[4,5,52,53] Cross-species infection of SFV from NHP to humans can occur as evidenced by serologic evidence of the virus in personnel exposed to NHP.[52] SFV seem to cause no clinical disease in NHP or humans. The virus has been detected in blood, oral mucosa, and feces,[52,53] and transmission likely occurs through biting, licking, sexual contact, and mucosal membrane exposure.[53] Although SFV seems to be nonpathogenic, caution still needs be present when working with NHP because of the potential for nonpathogenic viruses to become pathogenic once introduced into a new species.

Poxviruses

There are several types of pox virus (monkeypox, Yaba, smallpox, OrTeCa or benign epidermal monkeypox, and Molluscum contagiosum) that may have zoonotic potential.[4] Virus can be present in fluids and crusts from a lesion, respiratory secretions, or tissues.[4,5] Of the different pox viruses, monkeypox has the most clinical significance because of its wide range of reservoir hosts that can be responsible for human infections.[59]

Monkeypox is a virus endemic to central and western Africa that can cause fatal disease in children. Naturally acquired infections in animals have not been reported, and its natural animal reservoir remains unknown, although squirrels and rodents have been implicated.[59,60] In 2003, a monkeypox outbreak was reported in people that had come in contact with prairie dogs and other mammals.[59] The introduction of monkeypox into the United States was likely through shipment of small mammals (rope squirrels [*Funisciurus* spp], tree squirrels [*Heliosciurus* spp], Gambian giant rats [*Cricetomys* spp], brushtail porcupines [*Atherurus* spp], dormice [*Graphiurus* spp], and striped mice [*Hybomys* spp]) from Ghana to Texas.[61] Monkeypox was diagnosed using polymerase chain reaction in prairie dogs with clinical signs. The likely route of exposure was via respiratory secretions and direct mucocutaneous exposure in humans. Clinical symptoms in humans resemble smallpox infection but are generally less severe; symptoms include fever, malaise, maculopapular rash, and lymphadenopathy. Of these signs, lymphadenopathy is not characteristically seen in smallpox infection.[60] NHP have been proposed as a reservoir of the monkeypox virus because human infection has been reported after contact with infected NHPs.[4,5]

OrTeCa, or benign epidermal monkeypox, produces a mild disease in NHP, characterized by dermal lesions; humans develop lymphadenopathy and high fever.[4] Yaba poxvirus is an oncogenic virus that causes nodular lesions in humans but seems to regress in several months. Laboratory infection via a needle stick was reported with tumor resection being curative.[4] Molluscum contagiosum is a poxvirus that produces skin lesions in chimpanzees and humans.[4] Smallpox virus is considered eradicated by the World Health Organization; however, there are some concerns with the use of vector vaccine with vaccinia virus against other viruses (HIV) that may potentially expose primates to poxviruses.[4,5]

PARASITIC AGENTS

Parasites are common in both captive and wild NHP and can be present in both clinically normal and diseased animals. Personnel working with NHP are at risk of acquiring parasitic disease via contact with blood, feces, and tissue.[62–64] In addition, with the increase of international travel, immigrants, and immunocompromised people, parasitic infections need to be considered by physicians when consistent symptoms are present. A review of parasitic infections in humans in the laboratory setting was recently published.[62] Surveys of captive and wild populations of NHP that live near human populations have emphasized the potential impact of these organisms as zoonotic agents.[63,64] Potential exposure routes include accidental needle sticks, scratches, bite wounds, skin exposure, and vector-borne transmission.[62]

Potential intestinal parasites that may affect people working with NHP include *Strongyloides* spp, *Oesophagotomum apiostomum*, *Trichuris trichuria*, *Necator americanus*, *Ancylostoma duodenale*.[4,63,64] Mixed-species enclosures at zoologic institutions are a potential source of parasitic infection as some animals may serve as reservoirs of a parasite. In addition, vermin control in both zoologic institutions and laboratory settings is important because vermin may serve as not only reservoirs, but also vectors of parasites. *Baylisascaris procyonis*, the raccoon roundworm, which is a known zoonotic agent, has been reported in NHP with neurologic signs.[65]

Protozoal organisms that affect NHP also have the potential to cause zoonotic disease. Protozoal organisms can be transmitted via the fecal–oral route as well as via vectors.[66,67] *Plasmodium knowlesi*, a NHP protozoan transmitted by mosquitoes has been reported to cause disease and even death in humans.[66] Other *Plasmodium* spp that are present in NHP may have zoonotic potential and emphasizes the role of NHP as reservoirs.[67] NHP are carriers of several protozoal organisms in their feces such as *Giardia*, *Trichomonas*, and *Entoameba hystolitica*.[60,61] Although zoonotic infection with these organisms is not common, there is still potential for exposure.

Another protozoa with zoonotic potential is *Trypanosoma cruzi*, the causative agent of Chagas disease.[68] *T cruzi* infection in humans causes severe heart disease. Infection with *T cruzi* has been reported in both captive and free-ranging NHP.[6,68,69] The organism is primarily transmitted by the triatomine bug, although transfusion with infected blood can also lead to exposure.[69] The triatomine bug deposits fecal material with the parasite while taking a blood meal from the host. The animal or human then becomes infected when the fecal material enters the bite wound or crosses mucous membranes. NHP are not only affected by the disease, but also serve as reservoirs for the organism; other vermin species can also act as reservoirs.

Leishmaniasis, which is spread by sandflies, causes human infection in both a cutaneous and chronic visceral form and has also been reported in NHP.[4,5] A clinical case of *Leishmania* infection in a laboratory worker was caused by an accidental needle stick after handling an infected NHP.[70]

FUNGAL AGENTS

Mycotic infections are less common as zoonotic agents than bacteria and viruses. Some fungal infections may resemble tuberculosis because of granuloma formation and presence of bony lesions.[4,5] *Encephalitozoon bieneusi* was previously classified as a protozoan, but was recently reclassified as a zygomycete fungi by biochemical, phylogenetic, and genome analysis.[14] *E bieneusi* is an emerging pathogen present in healthy and immunocompromised macaques and can have significant impact on immunocompromised people, particularly in AIDS patients.[14] The organism causes chronic diarrhea and affects the biliary tract in AIDS patients. *Candida albicans*, mostly considered a opportunistic organism, can cause infection in the oral mucosa and genital mucosa, as well as generalized disease in immunocompromised individuals. The author has seen several cases of candidiasis in young animals with chronic diarrhea and prolonged antibiotic use. Although fungal zoonotic infections are not commonly reported, personnel should always be aware of potential exposure.

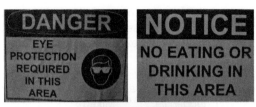

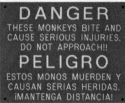

Fig. 6. Appropriate safety signs should be visible to staff and visitors.

PREVENTATIVE MEASURES/OCCUPATIONAL AND SAFETY GUIDELINES

Zoonotic diseases are an inherent risk for any person working with any animal, particularly NHP. The key to avoiding zoonotic infections is safety and prevention. Clear signs regarding safety rules need to be clearly posted for employees and visitors to see around the facility (**Fig. 6**). The US Centers for Disease Control and Prevention has published a set of guidelines when dealing with NHP.[71] Although the guidelines were intended for the Ebola-related cases in the United States, they provide important information regarding handling and quarantine of NHP.

Another important aspect in zoonotic disease prevention is disease surveillance. People who have a high level of exposure, either by occupational or recreational exposure, are of particular interest. Because these individuals are more likely to be exposed to pathogens than others, they may serve as potential carriers of an organism. Also, monitoring animal and human cases can serve as early signs of potential epizootics or epidemics.[72] Comparative medicine is the study of the anatomic, physiologic, and pathophysiologic processes across species, including humans.[73] In this field of medicine, emphasis is placed on infectious diseases, particularly on the host–agent interaction. Understanding these interactions may provide valuable information on zoonotic disease and cross-species infection of pathogens.

Diagnostic testing is essential to assess the health status, including the bacteriologic and viral status, of an animal or a colony. Bacterial culture for enteric pathogens in NHP is important in any facility and can provide important information, but false-negative results can occur.[74] Additional diagnostic tests such as polymerase chain reaction can provide further information in enteric pathogen infection. Viral testing is an essential tool in establishing the viral status of a NHP and can be performed using serologic and molecular assays. Numerous tests are available from several laboratories (**Table 1**). A complete post mortem examination provides valuable information regarding to the health status of a colony. Any animal that dies should have a complete necropsy and histopathology performed, as well as tissue archiving for possible additional testing.

Personal protective equipment is among the most significant, often underused aspect of disease prevention in a NHP facility. Level of protection is dictated by the species of NHP and organisms that the personnel may be exposed to, but basic use

Table 1
Diagnostic laboratories that provide simian viral testing

Name	Address	Tests Available
BioReliance Corp.	14920 Broshart Rd Rockville, MD 20850-3300 USA Telephone: 1-800 553 5372 Fax- 301-610-2590 Website: www.bioreliance.com	Herpes B, STLV-1, SIV, SRV, and foamy virus
Pathogen Detection Laboratory California National Primate Research Center	Road 98 & Hutchison University of California-Davis Davis, CA 95616 USA Telephone:530-752-4816 Website: http://pdl.primate.ucdavis.edu	SRV, SIV, STLV-1, SFV, measles, SV40
National B Virus Resource Center Viral Immunology Center Georgia State University	PO Box 4118 Atlanta, GA 30302-4118 USA Telephone: 404-413-6550 Fax: 404-413-6556; 404-413-6561	B virus or Cercophithecine herpesvirus 1

of mask, eye protection and gloves is of utmost importance. Any facility that houses NHP should have written guidelines regarding exposure to potential pathogens in place. These guidelines vary depending on the species of NHP housed.

SUMMARY

NHPs and humans share many similarities physiologically and anatomically. Because of this, NHP are excellent models for the study of human infectious disease; humans are also susceptible to viruses, bacteria, and parasites that affect NHP. Several factors such as work exposure, ecotourism, international travel, and the exotic pet trade play an important role in the development and maintenance of infectious diseases. Veterinarians must play a part in the education of the general population regarding zoonotic diseases and the impact these diseases may have on our world. Particular attention should be focused on zoonotic agents that have the potential to cross species, because they could lead to new diseases, epidemics, or epizootics. Veterinarians must work with professionals in the human medical field to increase the knowledge base of the host–pathogen interaction and provide answers regarding the behavior of these diseases.

ACKNOWLEDGMENTS

The author acknowledges the Caribbean Primate Research Center for their support and Drs Andres Mejia and Matt Kessler for their editorial assistance with this article.

REFERENCES

1. World Health Organization (WHO). Available at: www.who.int. Accessed December 12, 2010.
2. Woolhouse ME, Gowtage-Sequeria S. Host range and emerging and reemerging pathogens. Emerg Infect Dis 2005;11:1842–7.
3. Wolfe ND, Escalante AA, Karesh WB, et al. Wild primate populations in emerging infectious disease research: the missing link? Emerg Infect Dis 1998;4:149–58.
4. Fox JG. Laboratory animal medicine. 2nd edition. Amsterdam: Academic Press; 2002.

5. Bennett BT, Abee CR, Henrickson R. Nonhuman primates in biomedical research. San Diego: Academic Press; 1995.

6. Gardner MB, Luciw PA. Macaque models of human infectious disease. Ilar J 2008; 49:220–5.

7. Pedersen AB, Davies TJ. Cross-species pathogen transmission and disease emergence in primates. Ecohealth 2009;6:496–508.

8. Trevejo RT, Barr MC, Robinson RA. Important emerging bacterial zoonotic infections affecting the immunocompromised. Vet Res 2005;36:493–506.

9. Blancou J, Chomel BB, Belotto A, et al. Emerging or re-emerging bacterial zoonoses: factors of emergence, surveillance and control. Vet Res 2005;36:507–22.

10. World Health Organization. Xenotransplantation: guidance on infectious disease prevention and management. Available at: http://whqlibdoc.who.int/hq/1998/WHO_EMC_ZOO_98.1.pdf. Accessed May 12, 2011.

11. Une Y, Mori T. Tuberculosis as a zoonosis from a veterinary perspective. Comp Immunol Microbiol Infect Dis 2007;30:415–25.

12. US Centers for Disease Control and Prevention. Available at: www.cdc.gov/tb/statistics/default.htm. Accessed May 12, 2011.

13. Zumpe D, Silberman MS, Michael RP. Unusual outbreak of tuberculosis due to Mycobacterium bovis in a closed colony of rhesus monkeys (Macaca mulatta). Lab Anim Sci 1980;30:237–40.

14. Bailey C, Mansfield K. Emerging and reemerging infectious diseases of nonhuman primates in the laboratory setting. Vet Pathol 2010;47:462–81.

15. Fox JG. Laboratory animal medicine. San Diego: Academic Press; 2002.

16. Springer DA, Phillippi-Falkenstein K, Smith G. Retrospective analysis of wound characteristics and tetanus development in captive macaques. J Zoo Wildl Med 2009;40:95–102.

17. Kessler MJ, Berard JD, Rawlins RG, et al. Tetanus antibody titers and duration of immunity to clinical tetanus infections in free-ranging rhesus monkeys (Macaca mulatta). Am J Primatol 2006;68:725–31.

18. Chosewood LC, Wilson DE, Centers for Disease Control and Prevention (US), National Institutes of Health (US). Biosafety in microbiological and biomedical laboratories. 5th edition. Washington (DC): US Department of Health and Human Services, Public Health Service, Centers for Disease Control and Prevention, National Institutes of Health; 2009.

19. Banish LD, Sims R, Sack D, et al. Prevalence of shigellosis and other enteric pathogens in a zoologic collection of primates. J Am Vet Med Assoc 1993;203:126–32.

20. Sestak K, Merritt CK, Borda J, et al. Infectious agent and immune response characteristics of chronic enterocolitis in captive rhesus macaques. Infect Immun 2003;71:4079–86.

21. Tribe GW, Fleming MP. Biphasic enteritis in imported cynomolgus (Macaca fascicularis) monkeys infected with Shigella, Salmonella and Campylobacter species. Lab Anim 1983;17:65–9.

22. Nizeyi JB, Innocent RB, Erume J, et al. Campylobacteriosis, salmonellosis, and shigellosis in free-ranging human-habituated mountain gorillas of Uganda. J Wildl Dis 2001;37:239–44.

23. Kennedy FM, Astbury J, Needham JR, et al. Shigellosis due to occupational contact with non-human primates. Epidemiol Infect 1993;110:247–51.

24. DuPont HL, Levine MM, Hornick RB, et al. Inoculum size in shigellosis and implications for expected mode of transmission. J Infect Dis 1989;159:1126–8.

25. Niyogi SK. Shigellosis. J Microbiol 2005;43:133–43.

26. Barman S, Chatterjee S, Chowdhury G, et al. Plasmid-mediated streptomycin and sulfamethoxazole resistance in Shigella flexneri 3a. Int J Antimicrob Agents 2010;36: 348–51.

27. Caprioli A, Morabito S, Brugere H, et al. Enterohaemorrhagic Escherichia coli: emerging issues on virulence and modes of transmission. Vet Res 2005;36:289–311.

28. Pennington H. Escherichia coli O157. Lancet 23;376:1428–35.

29. US Centers for Disease Control and Prevention website. Campylobacter. Available at: http://www.cdc.gov/nczved/divisions/dfbmd/diseases/campylobacter/.   Accessed January 12, 2010.

30. Minette HP. Leptospirosis in primates other than man. Am J Trop Med Hyg 1966;15: 190–8.

31. Perolat P, Poingt JP, Vie JC, et al. Occurrence of severe leptospirosis in a breeding colony of squirrel monkeys. Am J Trop Med Hyg 1992;46:538–45.

32. Szonyi B, Agudelo-Florez P, Ramirez M, et al. An outbreak of severe leptospirosis in capuchin (Cebus) monkeys. Vet J 2011;188:237–9.

33. Matz-Rensing K, Floto A, Schrod A, et al. Epizootic of tularemia in an outdoor housed group of cynomolgus monkeys (Macaca fascicularis). Vet Pathol 2007;44:327–34.

34. Twenhafel NA, Alves DA, Purcell BK. Pathology of inhalational Francisella tularensis spp. tularensis SCHU S4 infection in African green monkeys (Chlorocebus aethiops). Vet Pathol 2009;46:698–706.

35. Nayar GP, Crawshaw GJ, Neufeld JL. Tularemia in a group of nonhuman primates. J Am Vet Med Assoc 1979;175:962–3.

36. Jones-Engel L, Engel GA, Schillaci MA, et al. Considering human-primate transmission of measles virus through the prism of risk analysis. Am J Primatol 2006;68:868–79.

37. Kondgen S, Kuhl H, N'Goran PK, et al. Pandemic human viruses cause decline of endangered great apes. Curr Biol 2008;18:260–4.

38. Willy ME, Woodward RA, Thornton VB, et al. Management of a measles outbreak among Old World nonhuman primates. Lab Anim Sci 1999;49:42–8.

39. Choi YK, Simon MA, Kim DY, et al. Fatal measles virus infection in Japanese macaques (Macaca fuscata). Vet Pathol 1999;36:594–600.

40. Huemer HP, Larcher C, Czedik-Eysenberg T, et al. Fatal infection of a pet monkey with Human herpesvirus. Emerg Infect Dis 2002;8:639–42.

41. Huff JL, Barry PA. B-virus (Cercopithecine herpesvirus 1) infection in humans and macaques: potential for zoonotic disease. Emerg Infect Dis 2003;9:246–50.

42. Ritz N, Curtis N, Buttery J, et al. Monkey bites in travelers: should we think of herpes B virus? Pediatr Emerg Care 2009;25:529–31.

43. Jensen K, Alvarado-Ramy F, Gonzalez-Martinez J, et al. B-virus and free-ranging macaques, Puerto Rico. Emerg Infect Dis 2004;10:494–6.

44. Schou S, Hansen AK. Marburg and Ebola virus infections in laboratory non-human primates: a literature review. Comp Med 2000;50:108–23.

45. Monath TP. Yellow fever: an update. Lancet Infect Dis 2001;1:11–20.

46. Rifakis PM, Benitez JA, De-la-Paz-Pineda J, et al. Epizootics of yellow fever in Venezuela (2004–2005): an emerging zoonotic disease. Ann N Y Acad Sci 2006; 1081:57–60.

47. Pavio N, Meng XJ, Renou C. Zoonotic hepatitis E: animal reservoirs and emerging risks. Vet Res 2010;41:46.

48. Institute of Laboratory Animal Resources (US). Committee on Occupational Safety and Health in Research Animal Facilities. Occupational health and safety in the care and use of research animals. Washington (DC): National Academy Press; 1997.

49. Meng XJ. Hepatitis E virus: animal reservoirs and zoonotic risk. Vet Microbiol 2010; 140:256–65.

50. Montali RJ, Connolly BM, Armstrong DL, et al. Pathology and immunohistochemistry of callitrichid hepatitis, an emerging disease of captive New World primates caused by lymphocytic choriomeningitis virus. Am J Pathol 1995;147:1441–9.

51. Khabbaz RF, Heneine W, George JR, et al. Brief report: infection of a laboratory worker with simian immunodeficiency virus. N Engl J Med 1994;330:172–7.

52. Khan AS. Simian foamy virus infection in humans: prevalence and management. Expert Rev Anti Infect Ther 2009;7:569–80.

53. Murphy HW, Miller M, Ramer J, et al. Implications of simian retroviruses for captive primate population management and the occupational safety of primate handlers. J Zoo Wildl Med 2006;37:219–33.

54. Zheng H, Wolfe ND, Sintasath DM, et al. Emergence of a novel and highly divergent HTLV-3 in a primate hunter in Cameroon. Virology 5;401:137-45.

55. Voevodin A, Samilchuk E, Schatzl H, et al. Interspecies transmission of macaque simian T-cell leukemia/lymphoma virus type 1 In baboons resulted in an outbreak of malignant lymphoma. J Virol 1996;70:1633–9.

56. Fowler ME, Miller RE. Zoo and wild animal medicine: current therapy. 6th edition. St. Louis: Saunders/Elsevier; 2008.

57. Lerche NW, Switzer WM, Yee JL, et al. Evidence of infection with simian type D retrovirus in persons occupationally exposed to nonhuman primates. J Virol 2001;75: 1783–9.

58. Song B, Javanbakht H, Perron M, et al. Retrovirus restriction by TRIM5alpha variants from Old World and New World primates. J Virol 2005;79:3930–7.

59. Guarner J, Johnson BJ, Paddock CD, et al. Monkeypox transmission and pathogenesis in prairie dogs. Emerg Infect Dis 2004;10:426–31.

60. Parker S, Nuara A, Buller RM, et al. Human monkeypox: an emerging zoonotic disease. Future Microbiol 2007;2:17–34.

61. Update: multistate outbreak of monkeypox—Illinois, Indiana, Kansas, Missouri, Ohio, and Wisconsin, 2003. MMWR Morb Mortal Wkly Rep 2003;52:642–6.

62. Herwaldt BL. Laboratory-acquired parasitic infections from accidental exposures. Clin Microbiol Rev 2001;14:659–88.

63. Munene E, Otsyula M, Mbaabu DA, et al. Helminth and protozoan gastrointestinal tract parasites in captive and wild-trapped African non-human primates. Vet Parasitol 1998;78:195–201.

64. Pourrut X, Diffo JL, Somo RM, et al. Prevalence of gastrointestinal parasites in primate bushmeat and pets in Cameroon. Vet Parasitol 10;175:187-91.

65. Sato H, Une Y, Kawakami S, et al. Fatal Baylisascaris larva migrans in a colony of Japanese macaques kept by a safari-style zoo in Japan. J Parasitol 2005;91:716–19.

66. Cox-Singh J, Davis TM, Lee KS, et al. Plasmodium knowlesi malaria in humans is widely distributed and potentially life threatening. Clin Infect Dis 2008;46:165–71.

67. Galinski MR, Barnwell JW. Monkey malaria kills four humans. Trends Parasitol 2009;25:200–4.

68. Carvalho CM, Andrade MC, Xavier SS, et al. Chronic Chagas' disease in rhesus monkeys (Macaca mulatta): evaluation of parasitemia, serology, electrocardiography, echocardiography, and radiology. Am J Trop Med Hyg 2003;68:683–91.

69. Pung OJ, Spratt J, Clark CG, et al. Trypanosoma cruzi infection of free-ranging lion-tailed macaques (Macaca silenus) and ring-tailed lemurs (Lemur catta) on St. Catherine's Island, Georgia, USA. J Zoo Wildl Med 1998;29:25–30.

70. Freedman DO, MacLean JD, Viloria JB. A case of laboratory acquired Leishmania donovani infection; evidence for primary lymphatic dissemination. Trans R Soc Trop Med Hyg 1987;81:118–9.
71. Update: Ebola-related filovirus infection in nonhuman primates and interim guidelines for handling nonhuman primates during transit and quarantine. MMWR Morb Mortal Wkly Rep 1990;39:22–4.
72. Wolfe ND, Dunavan CP, Diamond J. Origins of major human infectious diseases. Nature 2007;447:279–83.
73. Kahn LH. Confronting zoonoses, linking human and veterinary medicine. Emerg Infect Dis 2006;12:556–61.
74. Wang SM, Ma JC, Hao ZY, et al. Surveillance of shigellosis by real-time PCR suggests underestimation of shigellosis prevalence by culture-based methods in a population of rural China. J Infect 61:471-5.

Index

Note: Page numbers of article titles are in **boldface** type.

A

Acid-fast smears, for mycobacteriosis, 465
    in fish, 430–432
    in free-living birds, 494–495
Aeronomas spp., as zoonosis, associated with fish, 433
African hedgehogs, importation ban on, 542–543
Allergic pneumonitis, as zoonosis, in pet birds, 470–471
Allergies, skin, zoonoses and, in pet birds, 471
Amphibians, zoonoses associated with, **439–456**
    bacteria as, 440–449
        Chlamydia spp. as, 448–449
        Escherichia coli as, 447–448
        Mycobacterium spp. as, 446–447
        Salmonella spp. as, 446
        vancomycin-resistant Enterococci spp. as, 448
    fungi as, 452
    parasites as, 450–451
    prevention of, 440
    summary overview of, 439–440, 452
    viruses as, 451–452
Ancylostoma spp., as zoonosis, in nondomestic felids, 554
    in nonhuman primates, 569
Anthropozoonotic pathogens, 423
    viral, in nonhuman primates, 563–564
Antibiotic regimen, for chlamydiosis, in pet birds, 461
    for mycobacteriosis, in pet birds, 465
    for salmonellosis, in pet birds, 464
Antibody tests, for chlamydiosis, in pet birds, 460–461
    for rabies virus, 514
Antigen tests, for chlamydiosis, in pet birds, 460–461
Antimicrobial resistance, zoonoses and, associated with reptiles and amphibians, 443, 448
    in pet birds, 461, 464
    in poultry flock, 480
    multi-drug, 491
Arthropod-borne viruses, as zoonoses vector. See also specific virus, e.g., West Nile virus (WNV).
    in free-living birds, 497–499
    in poultry flock, 485–486
Aspergillus spp., as zoonosis, in pet birds, 468–469, 486

Vet Clin Exot Anim 14 (2011) 577–599
doi:10.1016/S1094-9194(11)00060-0
1094-9194/11/$ – see front matter © 2011 Elsevier Inc. All rights reserved.

vetexotic.theclinics.com

Avian influenza (AI), as zoonosis, in pet birds, 466–468
  in poultry flock, 483–485
 subtypes of, 483, 495
  pathogenic, 483, 495, 541
Avian paramyxoviruses (APMV), as zoonosis, in pet birds, 466–467

B

Bacteria, as zoonoses, associated with fish, 429–434
    Aeronomas spp. as, 433
    Edwardsiella spp. as, 433
    Erysipelothrix rhusiopathiae as, 431–432
    Mycobacterium spp. as, 429–432
    Salmonella spp. as, 433–434
    Streptococcus iniae as, 430–431
    Vibrio spp. as, 433
  associated with reptiles and amphibians, 440–449
    Chlamydia spp. as, 448–449
    Escherichia coli as, 447–448
    Mycobacterium spp. as, 446–447
    Salmonella spp. as, 440–446
    vancomycin-resistant *Enterococci* spp. as, 448
  in exotic pets, 533–539
    Campylobacter spp. as, 536–537
    Leptospira spp. as, 539
    Mycobacterium spp. as, 537–538
    Salmonella spp. as, 533–535
    Yersinia spp. as, 538–539
  in free-living birds, 492–495
    chlamydiosis as, 492–493
    Enterococcus spp. as, 492
    enteropathogens as, 493–494
    tuberculosis as, 494–495
  in nonhuman primates, 558–560
    Clostridium tetani as, 559–560
    enteric pathogens as, 560–563
    Mycobacterium spp. as, 558–559
  in pet birds, 457–466
    chlamydiosis as, 457–462
    mycobacteriosis as, 464–466
    other pathogens as, 466
    salmonellosis as, 462–464
  in poultry flock, 479–483
    Chlamydophila psittaci spp. as, 481–482
    Erysipelothrix rhusiopathiae as, 481
    food-borne, 480
    Mycobacterium avium subspecies *avium* as, 482–483
    Salmonella spp. as, 479–480
  in rabbits and rodents, **519–531**. See also *Rabbits; Rodents.*
  multidrug-resistant, 491
Bartonella spp., as zoonosis, in rodents, 523

Bats, rabies virus in, 508–510, 514
  bites and exposures from, 512–513
Baylisascaris procyonis, as zoonosis, in nonhuman primates, 569
  in raccoons, 552–553
Bearded dragons, zoonoses associated with, 445
Benign epidermal monkeypox, as zoonosis, in nonhuman primates, 568
Biosecurity of facilities, for free-living birds, 499–502
Birds, zoonoses related to, free-living, **491–505**. See also *Free-living birds.*
  pet, **457–476**. See also *Pet birds.*
  poultry, **477–490**. See also *Poultry flock.*
Bite wounds, rabies exposures and, 512–513
  risk of, in wildlife handlers, 492, 555
  zoonoses from, pet birds and, 471
    poultry flock and, 486
Blastomycosis, as zoonosis, in exotic pets, 541

C

Callitrichid hepatitis, as zoonosis, in nonhuman primates, 566
Campylobacter spp., as zoonosis, antimicrobial resistance and, 480
  in exotic pets, 536–537
  in free-living birds, 493
  in nonhuman primates, 562
  in pet birds, 466
  in poultry flock, 480
Candida spp., as zoonosis, in nonhuman primates, 569
  in pet birds, 468–469
Caracals, zoonoses carried by, 553–555
Carnivores, nondomestic, zoonoses carried by, **551–556**. See also *Felids; Procyonids.*
Cat scratch disease, 523
Cats, domestic, zoonoses carried by, charismatic nondomestic vs. See *Felids.*
    rabies virus as, 509
      bites and exposures from, 513
      vaccination for, 510–511
  ring-tailed, zoonoses carried by, 551
Cattle. See *Livestock.*
Cestodes, zoonoses and, associated with fish, 428
Chagas disease, as zoonosis, in nonhuman primates, 569
Cheyletiella spp., as zoonosis, in rabbits, 522
Chickens, backyard raising of. See *Poultry flock.*
  viral zoonoses in, clinical signs of, 483–485
Children, in developing countries, zoonosis risk for, 561
  poultry handling by, CDC recommendations for, 479–480
Chlamydia psittaci, as zoonosis, in free-living birds, 492–493
  in pet birds, 481–482
Chlamydia spp., as zoonosis, antimicrobial resistance and, 461
  associated with reptiles and amphibians, 448–449
  in pet birds, 457–462
Choana swabs, for chlamydiosis, in pet birds, 459–460
Climate change, global, zoonoses epidemics related to, 423–424
Clostridium perfringens, as zoonosis, in poultry flock, 480

Clostridium tetani, as zoonosis, in nonhuman primates, 559–560

Coat mundi, zoonoses carried by, 551

Coccidiomycosis, as zoonosis, in exotic pets, 541

Columbiform species, zoonoses of, 457. See also *Pet birds.*

Comparative medicine, for infectious agents, 570

Coxiella burnetti, as zoonosis, in rabbits, 522

Cryptococcus neoformans, as zoonosis, in poultry flock, 486

Cryptococcus spp., as zoonosis, in pet birds, 469

Cryptosporidium spp., as zoonosis, associated with fish, 428
    associated with reptiles and amphibians, 450–451
    in exotic pets, 544–545
    in pet birds, 469–470
    in poultry flock, 486–487
    in rabbits, 521

Cultures, for chlamydiosis, in pet birds, 459–460
  for *Mycobacterium avium* subspecies *avium,* in poultry flock, 482
  for salmonellosis, in pet birds, 463–464
  for zoonoses, in nonhuman primates, 570
    of pet birds skin lesions, 471

Cutaneous reactions. See *Skin lesions.*

D

Dermatologic conditions, with mycobacteriosis, in fish, 429–430
  with zoonoses, in pet birds, 471
    in rabbits and rodents, 527

Dermatophytosis, as zoonosis, in exotic pets, 539–541
    in nondomestic felids, 553–554
    in rabbits, 522–523

Direct fluorescent antibody (DFA), for rabies testing, 514

Disease surveillance, for handlers of nonhuman primates, 570

Disinfectants, for bacterial zoonoses, in free-living birds, 500–501
    in pet birds, 462, 464, 466
    in poultry flock, 478

Dogs, rabies virus in, 508–509
    bites and exposures from, 513
    vaccination for, 510–511

Domestic animals, nontraditional pets as. See also *Exotic animals/pets.*
    zoonoses carried by, 423, 551
  rabies virus in, bites and exposures from, 513
    prevalence and distribution of, 509–510
    vaccination for, 510–511
  zoonoses transmission between wildlife and, 499–500

Doxycycline, for chlamydiosis, in pet birds, 461

Drug resistance. See *Antimicrobial resistance.*

E

Eastern equine encephalitis (EEE), as zoonosis, in free-living birds, 497
    in poultry flock, 477, 485–486

Ebola virus, as zoonosis, 421
    in nonhuman primates, 565
    recent epidemics of, 421–422
Ectoparasites, zoonoses related to, in pet birds, 470
Education. See *Public health education.*
Edwardsiella spp., as zoonosis, associated with fish, 433
Encephalitis, as zoonosis, from free-living birds, 497, 499
Encephalitozoon bieneusi, as zoonosis, in nonhuman primates, 569
Encephalitozoon cuniculi, as zoonosis, in rabbits, 521
Enterococcus spp., as zoonosis, in free-living birds, 492–494
    in poultry flock, 480
    vancomycin-resistant, associated with reptiles and amphibians, 448
Enterohemorrhagic *Escherichia coli* (EHEC), as zoonosis, in nonhuman primates, 561
    in rabbits, 520–521
Enteropathogens, as zoonoses. See also *specific pathogen, e.g., Salmonella spp.*
    in free-living birds, 493–494
    in nondomestic felids, 554–555
    in nonhuman primates, 560–563
        Campylobacter spp. as, 562
        Escherichia coli as, 561–562
        leptospirosis as, 562–563
        morbidity and mortality with, 560
        Salmonella spp. as, 561
        Shigella spp. as, 561
        tularemia as, 563
        Yersinia enterocolitica as, 562
Epidemics, recent, of zoonoses, 421–422
Epidermophyton floccosum, as zoonosis, in exotic pets, 539
Erysipelothrix rhusiopathiae, as zoonosis, associated with fish, 431–432
    in poultry flock, 481
Escherichia coli, as zoonosis, associated with reptiles and amphibians, 447–448
    in free-living birds, 493
    in nonhuman primates, 561–562
    in pet birds, 466
    in poultry flock, 480
    in rabbits, enterohemorrhagic, 520–521
   serotypes of, 561–562
Euthanasia, of rabid animals, 511, 513–514
Exotic animals/pets, zoonoses carried by, **421–426**
    bacterial, 533–539
        Campylobacter spp. as, 536–537
        Leptospira spp. as, 539
        Mycobacterium spp. as, 537–538
        Salmonella spp. as, 533–535
        Yersinia spp. as, 538–539
    common companions, **533–549**. See also *Ferrets; Hedgehogs; Sugar gliders.*
    conclusions regarding, 424
    contributing factors of, 422–424
    fungal, 539–541
        dermatophytosis as, 539–541
        other diseases as, 541

legal implications of, 424
nondomestic, **551–556**. See also *Felids; Procyonids.*
parasitic, 543–545
  Cryptosporidium spp. as, 544–545
  giardiasis as, 544–545
  scabies as, 543
rabies virus as, 509
  bites and exposures from, 513
  vaccination for, 510–511
recent epidemics of, 421–422
summary overview of, 421, 423, 533, 545, 551
viral, 541–543
  foot and mouth virus as, 542–543
  influenza as, 541–542
wildlife species vs., 421–422

F

Favus, as zoonosis, in pet birds, 486
Felids, nondomestic, zoonoses carried by, **551–556**
    bite prevention for, 555
    dermatophytosis as, 553–554
    domestic vs. See *Cats.*
    enteric pathogens as, 554–555
    procyonids vs., 551–553
    species overview of, 551, 553, 555
Ferrets, zoonoses associated with, *Campylobacter* spp. as, 536–537
    Cryptosporidium spp. as, 544–545
    dermatophytosis as, 540
    Giardia spp. as, 544–545
    influenza A and B as, 541–542
      vaccination for, 542
    Leptospira spp. as, 539
    Mycobacterium spp. as, 537
    other fungal diseases as, 541
    rabies virus as, bites and exposures from, 513
      vaccination for, 510–511
    Salmonella spp. as, 535
    scabies as, 543
    Yersinia spp. as, 538–539
Filoviruses, as zoonosis, in nonhuman primates, 565
Fish, zoonoses associated with, **427–438**
    bacteria as, 429–434
      Aeronomas spp. as, 433
      Edwardsiella spp. as, 433
      Erysipelothrix rhusiopathiae as, 431–432
      Mycobacterium spp. as, 429–432
      Salmonella spp. as, 433–434
      Streptococcus iniae as, 430–431
      Vibrio spp. as, 433
    fungi as, 429

parasites as, 428
potential risks of, 427
prevention of, 434
protozoa as, 428
taxonomic group of, 427
Flukes, zoonoses and, associated with fish, 428
Fluroroquinolones, resistance to, in poultry flock, 480
Food sources, exotic pet, of *Salmonella* spp., 535
    fish, of protozoa and parasites, 428
    nonhuman primates, of zoonoses, 562, 566
    poultry, of bacterial zoonoses, 479–480
    reptile, of *Salmonella* spp., 446
Foot and mouth virus, as zoonosis, in exotic pets, 542–543
Foxes, rabies virus in, 507, 509
    bites and exposures from, 512–513
Francisella tularensis, as zoonosis, in nonhuman primates, 563
    in rabbits, 520
    in rodents, 520
Free-living birds, public health concerns associated with, **491–505**
    bacterial, 492–495
        chlamydiosis as, 492–493
        Enterococcus spp. as, 492
        enteropathogens as, 493–494
        tuberculosis as, 494–495
    biosecurity of facilities and, 499–502
    exposure prevention protocols for, 499–502
    health screening protocols for, 500
    introduction to, 491–492
    occupational injury risk for, 492
    personnel management and, 501–502
    summary overview of, 502
    viral, 495–499
        arboviruses as, 497–499
        influenza as, 495–497
        West Nile virus as, 497–499
Fungi, as zoonoses, associated with fish, 429
    associated with reptiles and amphibians, 452
    in exotic pets, 539–541
        dermatophytosis as, 539–541
        other diseases as, 541
    in nondomestic felids, 553–554
    in nonhuman primates, 569
    in pet birds, 468–469
    in poultry flock, 486

G

Game birds, public health concerns associated with care of. See *Free-living birds.*
Giardia spp., as zoonosis, in exotic pets, 544–545
    in pet birds, 469–470
Gorillas, retroviral diseases in, 567

Gram-negative bacteria, as zoonosis. See also *Salmonella spp.*
  associated with fish, 433
  in pet birds, 466
  in rodents, 523
Granulomas, with mycobacteriosis, 430–432

H

H1N1 influenza, as zoonosis, 484
  in ferrets, 541–542
  in free-living birds, 495–496
H3N2 influenza, as zoonosis, 484, 495–496
H5N1 influenza, as zoonosis, 483, 495–496
H7N7 influenza, as zoonosis, 483–484, 495–496
Habitats, natural vs. urban, zoonoses potential related to, 423, 491–492, 533, 557, 560
Handling protocols, for free-living birds, 492, 501–502
  for nonhuman primates, 570–571
  for poultry, by children, 479–480
  for wildlife, 499–502
Hantavirus pulmonary syndrome (HPS), 525
Hantaviruses, as zoonosis, in rodents, 525
Health care professionals, legal responsibilities of, regarding rabies prevention, 511–512
  regarding zoonoses, 424
Health screening protocols, for free-living birds, 500
Hedgehogs, zoonoses associated with, *Cryptosporidium* spp. as, 544–545
  dermatophytosis as, 540–541
  foot and mouth virus as, 542–543
  Mycobacterium spp. as, 537–538
  Salmonella spp. as, 535
  Yersinia spp. as, 538–539
Hepatitis virus, as zoonosis, in nonhuman primates, 565–566
    callitrichid, 566
Herpesviruses, as zoonosis, in nonhuman primates, 563–565, 571
High efficiency particulate air (HEPA) filter, for zoonoses prevention, in free-living bird handlers, 500–501
Hippocampus erectus, coelomic granulomas in, 430–431
Histoplasmosis capsulatum, as zoonosis, in poultry flock, 486
Histoplasmosis spp., as zoonosis, in pet birds, 469
Hookworms, as zoonosis, in nondomestic felids, 554–555
Horses, rabies virus in, 509–510
HPAI (highly pathogenic avian influenza), as zoonosis, in free-living birds, 496–497
  in poultry flocks, 483–484
Human diploid cell vaccine, as prophylaxis, for bites from rabid animals, 513–514
Human populations, animal transmission of infectious agents to, 421, 423. See also *Zoonoses.*
  increases in, zoonoses epidemics related to, 423, 491, 533
  rabies exposures of, 512–514
    bite vs. nonbite, 512
    diagnosis of, 514

from non-vector wildlife species, 513
    medical care and consultation for, 512–513
    post-exposure prophylaxis for, 513–514
    pre-exposure prophylaxis for, 501, 512
  transmission of infectious agents to animals by, 423
    viral, 563–564
Human rabies immune globulin (HRIG), as prophylaxis, for bites from rabid animals, 513–514
Husbandry guidelines, for zoonoses prevention, in free-living birds, 500–501
    in pet birds, 461–462, 464–466, 468
    in poultry flock, 477–479
Hypersensitivities, in pet birds, zoonoses and, 470–471
Hypersensitivity pneumonitis (HP), as zoonosis, in pet birds, 470–471

    I

Iguanas, green, zoonoses associated with, 445
Immunizations. See *Vaccinations.*
Immunocompromised humans, zoonoses in, 464–465, 482, 569
    prevention of, 440, 479
Immunohistochemistry (IHC), for West Nile virus, in free-living birds, 499
Imovax, as prophylaxis, for bites from rabid animals, 513–514
Importation bans, on African hedgehogs, 542–543
IMRAB 3, as rabies vaccination, 510–511
IMRAB Large Animal, as rabies vaccination, 511
Incubation period, for infectious diseases, 500
    for influenza viruses, 541
    for rabies virus, 508
    for *Salmonella* spp., 534
Infectious agents, animal transmission to humans, 421, 423, 477. See also *Zoonoses.*
    comparative medicine for, 570
    human transmission to animals, 423
      viral, 563–564
Influenza A, as zoonosis, in exotic pets, 541–542
    in free-living birds, 495–497
    in pet birds, 466–468
Influenza B, as zoonosis, in ferrets, 541–542
Influenza C, as zoonosis, in exotic pets, 541
Influenza viruses, as zoonoses, in birds. See *Avian influenza (AI).*
    in exotic pets, 541–542
    clinical signs of, 542
    subtypes of, 483, 495, 541
Interstate regulation, of turtles, by FDA, 442–443
Isolation, as biosecurity, for free-living birds, 500
    for chlamydiosis, in pet birds, 461–462

    J

Jaguars, zoonoses carried by, 553–555

K

Kinkajous, zoonoses carried by, 551–552
   Baylisascaris procyonis as, 552–553
Klebsiella spp., as zoonosis, in pet birds, 466

L

Legal implications, of zoonoses, 424, 478–479
Leishmaniasis, as zoonosis, in nonhuman primates, 569
Lentivirus, as zoonosis, in nonhuman primates, 567
Leopards, zoonoses carried by, 553–555
Leptospira spp., as zoonosis, in exotic pets, 539
   in nonhuman primates, 562–563
   in rodents, 523
Lesions, dermatologic. See *Skin lesions.*
  on internal organs, with parasite infestations, 428
   with West Nile virus, 498–499
  on joints, with mycobacteriosis, 429–430
Lions, zoonoses carried by, charismatic vs. mountain species, 553–555
Listeria monocytogenes, as zoonosis, in poultry flock, 480
Livestock, rabies virus in, clinical signs and progression of, 508–509
   prevalence and distribution of, 509–510
   vaccination for, 510–511
LPAI (low pathogenic avian influenza), as zoonosis, in free-living birds, 496
   in poultry flocks, 483–484
Lymphocytic choriomeningitis virus (LCMV), as zoonosis, in rodents, 525–526

M

Margay, zoonoses carried by, 553–555
Measles, as zoonosis, in nonhuman primates, 563, 571
Medical waste disposal, for zoonoses prevention, in free-living birds, 501
Meningitis, as zoonosis, in pet birds, 469
Microsporum canis, as zoonosis, in nondomestic felids, 553–554
   in rabbits, 522
Microsporum gallinae, as zoonosis, in pet birds, 486
Microsporum spp., as zoonosis, in exotic pets, 539–541
Mites, as zoonoses vector, associated with reptiles and amphibians, 450–451
   in exotic pets, 543
   in pet birds, 470
   in poultry flock, 486
   in rabbits and rodents, 522, 526–527
Molluscum contagiosum, as zoonosis, in nonhuman primates, 568
Monkeypox virus, as zoonosis, 421, 423
   in nonhuman primates, 568
   in rodents, 526
   recent epidemics of, 421–422
Mosquitoes, as zoonoses vector, in nonhuman primates, 569
   in pet birds, 468
Mycobacterium avium subspecies *avium,* as zoonosis, in free-living birds, 494–495
   in poultry flock, 482–483

Mycobacterium avium-intracellulare complex (MAC), as zoonosis, in free-living birds, 494
Mycobacterium spp., as zoonosis, associated with fish, 429–432
    associated with reptiles and amphibians, 446–447
    in exotic pets, 537–538
    in free-living birds, 494
    in nonhuman primates, 558–559
    in pet birds, 464–466
    transmission and prevention of, 538
Mycobacterium tuberculosis. See *Tuberculosis.*
Mycoses. See *Fungi.*

N

Negri bodies, rabies virus replication and, 508
Nematodes, zoonoses and, associated with fish, 428
    in raccoons, 552–553
Neurologic signs, of West Nile virus, in free-living birds, 497–499
Newcastle disease virus (NDV), as zoonosis, in pet birds, 466–467
    in poultry flock, 484–485
Nondomestic carnivores, zoonoses carried by, **551–556**. See also *Felids; Procyonids.*
Nonhuman primates (NHPs), zoonotic diseases of, **557–575**
    bacterial, 558–560
        Clostridium tetani as, 559–560
        enteric pathogens as, 560–563
        Mycobacterium spp. as, 558–559
    enteric pathogens and, 560–563
        Campylobacter spp. as, 562
        Escherichia coli as, 561–562
        leptospirosis as, 562–563
        morbidity and mortality with, 560
        Salmonella spp. as, 561
        Shigella spp. as, 561
        tularemia as, 563
        Yersinia enterocolitica as, 562
    fungal, 569
    parasitic, 568–569
    potential impact of, 558
    prevention of, 559–560, 562, 570–571
    summary overview of, 557, 571
    viral, 563–568
        anthropozoonotic potential vs., 563–564
        callitrichid hepatitis as, 566
        filoviruses as, 565
        hepatitis virus as, 565–566
        herpesviruses as, 563–565, 571
        measles as, 563, 571
        paramyxoviruses as, 563
        poxviruses as, 568
        retroviral diseases as, 566–568
        simian retrovirus as, 567, 571

SIV as, 567, 571
spumavirus as, 568
STLV as, 566–567, 571
yellow fever as, 565
Nontraditional pets. See *Exotic animals/pets.*
Non-vector wildlife species, zoonoses carried by, 513
Nutrition, for zoonoses prevention, in poultry flock, 478–479
  zoonoses related to. See *Food sources.*

O

Occupational health and safety plans, for handlers, of free-living birds, 492, 501–502
  of nonhuman primates, 570–571
Occupational injury risk, of wildlife handlers, 492
    prevention of, 499–502
  with nonhuman primates, 569–570
Ocelot, zoonoses carried by, 553–555
Olingos, zoonoses carried by, 551
"One Health," 421, 424. See also *Zoonoses.*
Oral rabies vaccination (ORV), of wildlife, 512
Ornithonyssus bacoti, as zoonosis, in rodents, 526–527
OrTeCa virus, as zoonosis, in nonhuman primates, 568
Owls, public health concerns associated with care of. See *Free-living birds.*
  screech, West Nile virus signs in, 497–498

P

Paramyxoviruses (PMV), as zoonosis, in nonhuman primates, 563
  in pet birds, 466–467
Parasites, as zoonoses, associated with fish, 428
    associated with reptiles and amphibians, 450–451
  in exotic pets, 543–545
    Cryptosporidium spp. as, 544–545
    giardiasis as, 544–545
    scabies as, 543
  in nondomestic felids, 554–555
  in nonhuman primates, 568–569
  in pet birds, 469–470
  in poultry flock, 486–487
  in rabbits and rodents, **519–531**. See also *Rabbits; Rodents.*
  in raccoons, 552–553
Passerine species, zoonoses of, 457. See also *Pet birds.*
Pasteurella spp., as zoonosis, in pet birds, 466
  in rabbits, 521–522
Pentastomes, as zoonosis, associated with reptiles and amphibians, 450
Personal protective equipment (PPE), in zoonoses prevention, with fish, 434
  with free-living birds, 500–502
  with nonhuman primates, 559–560, 570–571
  with pet birds, 462, 464
Personnel management, for free-living bird facilities, 501–502
Pet birds, zoonoses of, **457–476**

bacterial, 457–466
  chlamydiosis as, 457–462
  mycobacteriosis as, 464–466
  other pathogens as, 466
  salmonellosis as, 462–464
dermatologic conditions and, 471
fungal, 468–469
hypersensitivities and, 470–471
parasitic, 469–470
prevention of, 461–462, 464–466, 468
summary overview of, 457, 471
viral, 466–468
  influenza as, 467–468
  Newcastle disease virus as, 466–467
  West Nile virus as, 468
Pet ownership, zoonoses epidemics related to, 423. See also *Exotic animals/pets.*
Physicians, legal responsibilities of, regarding zoonoses, 424
Plasmodium spp., as zoonosis, in nonhuman primates, 569
Pneumonitis, allergic/hypersensitivity, as zoonosis, in pet birds, 470–471
Polymerase chain reaction (PCR), for chlamydiosis, in pet birds, 460–461
  for West Nile virus, in free-living birds, 499
  for zoonoses, in nonhuman primates, 570
Post-exposure prophylaxis, for rabies virus, 513–514
Potbellied pigs, rabies virus in, 508–509
Poultry flock, backyard, zoonoses and, **477–490**
  antimicrobial resistance in, 480
  bacterial, 479–483
    Chlamydophila psittaci spp. as, 481–482
    Erysipelothrix rhusiopathiae as, 481
    food-borne, 480
    Mycobacterium avium subspecies *avium* as, 482–483
    Salmonella spp. as, 479–480
  commercial flocks vs., 477
  fungal, 486
  parasitic, 486–487
  prevalence of, 477
  prevention recommendations for, 477–479
  summary overview of, 477, 487
  viral, 483–486
    arthropod-borne, 485–486
    avian influenza as, 483–484
    clinical signs of, 483–485
    Newcastle disease as, 484–485
Poxviruses, as zoonosis, in nonhuman primates, 568
Pre-exposure prophylaxis, for rabies virus, 501, 512
Prevention of zoonoses, associated with fish, 434
  associated with reptiles and amphibians, 440
  in exotic pets, *Salmonella* spp. and, 535
  in free-living birds, 499–502
  in nonhuman primates, 559–560, 562, 570–571
  in pet birds, 461–462, 464–466, 468

in poultry flock, 477–479
in wildlife, 553, 555
legal responsibilities for, 424
Primates, human. See *Human populations.*
nonhuman. See *Nonhuman primates (NHPs).*
Procyonids, zoonoses carried by, **551–556**
    Baylisascaris procyonis as, 552–553
    bite prevention for, 555
    nondomestic felids vs., 553–555
    species overview of, 551, 555
Protozoa, as zoonosis, associated with fish, 428
    in nonhuman primates, 569
Psittacine species, zoonoses of, 457. See also *Pet birds.*
Public health, infectious disease transmission as concern for. See *Zoonoses; specific species, e.g., Free-living birds.*
Public health education, on rabies virus, 511–512
    on zoonoses, 424
    on zoonoses prevention. See *Prevention of zoonoses.*
Purified chick embryo cell vaccine, as prophylaxis, for bites from rabid animals, 513–514

Q

Q fever, as zoonosis, in rabbits, 522
Quarantine, as biosecurity, for free-living birds, 500
    for chlamydiosis, in pet birds, 461–462

R

RabAvert, as prophylaxis, for bites from rabid animals, 513–514
Rabbits, zoonoses of, **519–531**
    Cheyletiella spp. as, 522
    Coxiella burnetti as, 522
    Cryptosporidium spp. as, 521
    dermatophytosis as, 522–523
    Encephalitozoon cuniculi as, 521
    enterohemorrhagic *Escherichia coli* as, 520–521
    Francisella tularensis as, 520
    introduction to, 519
    Pasteurella spp. as, 521–522
    summary overview of, 527
    Yersinia pestis as, 519–520
Rabies Control, web site for, 511
Rabies Management Program, National, 512
Rabies vaccination, of humans, pre-exposure, 501, 512
    of livestock and pets, 510–511
    of wildlife, 511
        oral, 512
Rabies virus, **507–518**
    clinical signs and progression of, 508–509
    euthanasia indications for, 511, 513–514

genus of, 507
human exposure to, 512–514
  bite vs. nonbite, 512
  diagnosis of, 514
  from non-vector wildlife species, 513
  medical care and consultation for, 512–513
  post-exposure prophylaxis for, 513–514
  pre-exposure prophylaxis for, 501, 512
pathogenesis of, 508
prevalence and distribution of, in Canada, 510
  in Mexico, 510
  in US animals, 509–510
prevention of, 510–512
  public education for, 511–512
  vaccination for, human pre-exposure, 501, 512
    in livestock and pets, 510–511
    in wildlife, 512
testing for, 514
variants of, 507–508
Raboral V-RG, as rabies vaccination, 511
Raccoons, zoonoses carried by, *Baylisascaris procyonis* as, 552–553, 569
  minor pathogens as, 552
  rabies virus as, 507, 509
    bites and exposures from, 512–513
  species overview of, 551, 555
Raptors, public health concerns associated with care of. See *Free-living birds.*
Rat bite fever (RBF), as zoonosis, in rodents, 524
Rat-mite dermatitis, 527
Rat-mite vector, of *Ornithonyssus bacoti,* in rodents, 526–527
Reptile-associated salmonellosis (RAS), 443–444
Reptiles, zoonoses associated with, **439–456**
  bacteria as, 440–449
    Chlamydia spp. as, 448–449
    Escherichia coli as, 447–448
    Mycobacterium spp. as, 446–447
    Salmonella spp. as, 440–446
      classification reorganization and, 440–441
      food sources of, 446
      history of, 441
      reptile species and, 443–446
      serotypes of, 440–441, 443–444
      turtles and, 441–443
    vancomycin-resistant *Enterococci* spp. as, 448
  fungi as, 452
  parasites as, 450–451
  prevention of, 440
  summary overview of, 439–440, 452
  viruses as, 451–452
Reservoirs, of zoonoses, rodents as, **519–531**. See also *Rodents.*
  vermin as, 569
  wildlife species as, 421–423, 491, 500, 552

Retroviral diseases, as zoonoses, in nonhuman primates, 566–568
    diagnostic tests for, 570–571
    simian retrovirus as, 567, 571
    SIV as, 567, 571
    spumavirus as, 568
    STLV as, 566–567, 571
Reverse-transcriptase PCR (RT-PCR), for rabies testing, 514
RFFIT serologic test, for rabies virus antibody, 514
Rhesus macaque, zoonosis associated with, herpesviruses as, 563–564
    shigellosis as, 561
Rickettsia akari, as zoonosis, in rodents, 524
Rickettsia typhi, as zoonosis, in rodents, 524–525
Ring-tailed cats, zoonoses carried by, 551
Rodents, zoonoses of, **519–531**
    Bartonella spp. as, 523
    Francisella tularensis as, 520
    hantaviruses as, 525
    introduction to, 519
    Leptospira spp. as, 523
    lymphocytic choriomeningitis virus as, 525–526
    monkeypox virus as, 526
    nonhuman primates and, 562
    Ornithonyssus bacoti as, 526–527
    rabies virus as, bites and exposures from, 513
    rat-mite vector of, 526–527
    Rickettsia akari as, 524
    Rickettsia typhi as, 524–525
    Salmonella spp. as, 523–524
    Streptobacillus moniliformis as, 524
    summary overview of, 527
    Yersinia pestis as, 519–520

S

Safety protocols. See *Handling protocols; Occupational health and safety plans.*
Safety signs, for handlers, of nonhuman primates, 570
Salmonella spp., as zoonosis, 421
    antimicrobial resistance and, 443, 464
    associated with amphibians, 446
    associated with fish, 433–434
    associated with reptiles, 440–446
      classification reorganization and, 440–441
      food sources of, 446
      history of, 441
      reptile species and, 443–446
      turtles and, 441–443
    clinical signs of, 534
    genus of, 533–534
    in exotic pets, 533–535
    in free-living birds, 493
    in nondomestic felids, 554–555

in nonhuman primates, 561
in pet birds, 462–464
in poultry flock, 479–480
in rodents, 523–524
prevalence of, 534
recent epidemics of, 421–422
transmission and prevention of, 535
serotypes of, atypical, 443–444
reclassification of, 440–441
Sandflies, as zoonoses vector, in nonhuman primates, 569
Scabies, as zoonosis, in exotic pets, 543
Screech owl, West Nile virus signs in, 497–498
Serotypes, of avian influenza, 483, 495
pathogenic subtypes, 483, 495, 541
of Escherichia coli, 561–562
of Salmonella spp., 440–441, 443
atypical, 443–444
Servals, zoonoses carried by, 553–555
Sheep, rabies virus in, 509–510
vaccination for, 510–511
Shigella spp., as zoonosis, in nonhuman primates, 561
Simian foamy viruses (SFV), as zoonosis, in nonhuman primates, 568, 571
Simian retrovirus (SRV), as zoonosis, in nonhuman primates, 567, 571
SIV, as zoonosis, in nonhuman primates, 567, 571
Skin allergies, zoonoses and, in pet birds, 471
Skin lesions, in fish, with mycobacteriosis, 429–430
in pet birds, cultures for zoonoses, 471
rat-mites causing, 527
Skin tests, for tuberculosis, 559
Skunks, rabies virus in, 507–509
bites and exposures from, 512–513
Smallpox, as zoonosis, in nonhuman primates, 568
Snake mites, zoonoses and, associated with reptiles and amphibians, 451
Snakes, zoonoses associated with, 441, 445
Spumavirus, as zoonosis, in nonhuman primates, 568
Standard Precautions, for Zoonotic Disease Prevention, 424, 479. See also Personal protective equipment (PPE).
Staphylococcus spp., as zoonosis, in poultry flock, 480
STLV, as zoonosis, in nonhuman primates, 566–567, 571
Streptobacillus moniliformis, as zoonosis, in rodents, 524
Streptococcus iniae, as zoonosis, associated with fish, 430–431
Streptococcus spp., as zoonosis, in poultry flock, 480
Sudden Acute Respiratory Syndrome (SARS), as zoonosis, 421
Sugar gliders, zoonoses associated with, Giardia spp. as, 544–545
Salmonella spp. as, 535
Surveillance, disease, for handlers of nonhuman primates, 570

T

Tetanus, as zoonosis, in nonhuman primates, 559–560
Thogotovirus, as zoonosis, in exotic pets, 541

Ticks, as zoonoses vector, associated with reptiles and amphibians, 450–451
    in rabbits, 522
Tigers, zoonoses carried by, 553–555
Toxocara cati, as zoonosis, in nondomestic felids, 554
Toxoplasma gondii, as zoonosis, in nondomestic felids, 555
    in poultry flock, 486–487
Trematodes, zoonoses and, associated with fish, 428
Trichophyton mentagrophytes, as zoonosis, in rabbits, 522–523
Trichophyton spp., as zoonosis, in exotic pets, 539–541
Trypanosoma cruzi, as zoonosis, in nonhuman primates, 569
Tuberculosis, as zoonosis, avian, free-living birds and, 494–495
        pet birds and, 465
    in nonhuman primates, 558–559
    tests for, 559
Tularemia. See *Francisella tularensis.*
Turtle-associated salmonellosis, in humans, 441–443
Turtles, interstate regulation of, by FDA, 442–443

V

Vaccinations, for arthropod-born viruses, in poultry flock, 485–486
    for influenza, in ferrets, 542
    for rabies virus, human post-exposure, 513–514
        human pre-exposure, 501, 512
        in livestock and pets, 510–511
        in wildlife, 511–512
    for tetanus, in nonhuman primates, 559–560
Vancomycin-resistant *Enterococci* spp., as zoonosis, associated with reptiles and amphibians, 448
Vectors, for zoonoses, associated with reptiles and amphibians, 450–451
        in exotic pets, 543
        in free-living birds, 497–499
        in nonhuman primates, 569
        in pet birds, 468, 470
        in poultry flock, 485–486
        in rabbits and rodents, 522, 526–527
        non-vector wildlife species vs., 513
Vermin, as zoonosis reservoir, 569
Veterinarians, legal responsibilities of, regarding rabies prevention, 511–512
        regarding zoonoses, 424
Vibrio spp., as zoonosis, associated with fish, 433
Viral assay tests, for zoonoses, in nonhuman primates, 570–571
Viruses, as zoonoses, associated with reptiles and amphibians, 451–452
            West Nile virus as, 439, 452
        in exotic pets, 541–543
            foot and mouth virus as, 542–543
            influenza as, 541–542
        in free-living birds, 495–499
            arboviruses as, 497–499
            influenza as, 495–497

West Nile virus as, 497–499
in nonhuman primates, 563–568
    anthropozoonotic potential vs., 563–564
    callitrichid hepatitis as, 566
    filoviruses as, 565
    hepatitis virus as, 565–566
    herpesviruses as, 563–565, 571
    measles as, 563, 571
    paramyxoviruses as, 563
    poxviruses as, 568
    retroviral diseases as, 566–568
    simian retrovirus as, 567, 571
    SIV as, 567, 571
    spumavirus as, 568
    STLV as, 566–567, 571
    yellow fever as, 565
in pet birds, 466–468
    influenza as, 467–468
    Newcastle disease virus as, 466–467
    West Nile virus as, 468
in poultry flock, 483–486
    arthropod-borne, 485–486
    avian influenza as, 483–484
    Newcastle disease as, 484–485
in rabbits and rodents, **519–531**. See also *Rabbits; Rodents.*
rabies as, **507–518**. See also *Rabies virus.*

W

Waterfowl, public health concerns associated with care of. See *Free-living birds.*
West Nile virus (WNV), as zoonosis, 424
    associated with reptiles and amphibians, 439, 452
    in free-living birds, 497–499
    in pet birds, 466, 468
    in poultry flock, 485–486
    clinical signs of, in screech owl, 497–498
Western equine encephalitis (WEE), as zoonosis, in free-living birds, 497
    in poultry flock, 477, 485–486
Wildlife species, zoonoses carried by, 421–423, 491, 500, 552. See also *specific species, e.g., Felids.*
    rabies virus as, bites and exposures from, 512–513
        from non-vector species, 513
        prevalence and distribution of, 509–510
        vaccination for, 511–512
    zoonoses transmission between domestic species and, 499–500
Wound care, for bites from rabid animals, 513
    for injuries, from free-living birds, 492
Wounds, from bites. See *Bite wounds.*
    occupational types of, of wildlife handlers, 492, 495, 555
        with nonhuman primates, 569–570

Y

Yaba virus, as zoonosis, in nonhuman primates, 568
Yellow fever, as zoonosis, in nonhuman primates, 565
Yersinia enterocolitica, as zoonosis, in nonhuman primates, 562
Yersinia pestis, as zoonosis, in exotic pets, 538
       in rabbits, 519–520
       in rodents, 519–520
Yersinia pseudotuberculosis, as zoonosis, in exotic pets, 538–539
Yersinia spp., as zoonosis, in exotic pets, 538–539
       in pet birds, 466

Z

Zooanthroponotic pathogens, 423
   nonhuman primates and, 563–564
Zoonoses, associated with fish, **427–438**
       bacteria as, 429–434
           Aeronomas spp. as, 433
           Edwardsiella spp. as, 433
           Erysipelothrix rhusiopathiae as, 431–432
           Mycobacterium spp. as, 429–432
           Salmonella spp. as, 433–434
           Streptococcus iniae as, 430–431
           Vibrio spp. as, 433
       fungi as, 429
       parasites as, 428
       potential risks of, 427
       prevention of, 434
       protozoa as, 428
       taxonomic group of, 427
   associated with reptiles and amphibians, **439–456**
       bacteria as, 440–449
           Chlamydia spp. as, 448–449
           Escherichia coli as, 447–448
           Mycobacterium spp. as, 446–447
           Salmonella spp. as, 440–446
           vancomycin-resistant *Enterococci* spp. as, 448
       fungi as, 452
       parasites as, 450–451
       prevention of, 440
       summary overview of, 439–440, 452
       viruses as, 451–452
   definition of, 421, 423, 477
   incidence of, habitat intermingling and, 491–492
   multidrug-resistant, 491
   of common pet birds, **457–476**
       bacterial, 457–466
           chlamydiosis as, 457–462
           mycobacteriosis as, 464–466
           other pathogens as, 466

salmonellosis as, 462–464
dermatologic conditions and, 471
fungal, 468–469
hypersensitivities and, 470–471
parasitic, 469–470
summary overview of, 457, 471
viral, 466–468
influenza as, 467–468
Newcastle disease virus as, 466–467
West Nile virus as, 468
of exotic pets, **421–426**
bacterial, 533–539
Campylobacter spp. as, 536–537
Leptospira spp. as, 539
Mycobacterium spp. as, 537–538
Salmonella spp. as, 533–535
Yersinia spp. as, 538–539
common, **533–549**. See also *Ferrets; Hedgehogs; Sugar gliders.*
conclusions regarding, 424
contributing factors of, 422–424
fungal, 539–541
dermatophytosis as, 539–541
other diseases as, 541
legal implications of, 424
parasitic, 543–545
Cryptosporidium spp. as, 544–545
giardiasis as, 544–545
scabies as, 543
recent epidemics of, 421–422
summary overview of, 421, 533, 545
viral, 541–543
foot and mouth virus as, 542–543
influenza as, 541–542
wildlife species vs., 421–422
of free-living birds, **491–505**
bacterial, 492–495
chlamydiosis as, 492–493
Enterococcus spp. as, 492
enteropathogens as, 493–494
tuberculosis as, 494–495
biosecurity of facilities and, 499–502
exposure prevention protocols for, 499–502
introduction to, 491–492
occupational injury risk for, 492
personnel management and, 501–502
summary overview of, 502
viral, 495–499
arboviruses as, 497–499
influenza as, 495–497
West Nile virus as, 497–499
of nonhuman primates, **557–575**

bacterial, 558–560
  Clostridium tetani as, 559–560
  enteric pathogens as, 560–563
  Mycobacterium spp. as, 558–559
enteric pathogens and, 560–563
  Campylobacter spp. as, 562
  Escherichia coli as, 561–562
  leptospirosis as, 562–563
  morbidity and mortality with, 560
  Salmonella spp. as, 561
  Shigella spp. as, 561
  tularemia as, 563
  Yersinia enterocolitica as, 562
fungal, 569
parasitic, 568–569
potential impact of, 558
prevention of, 559–560, 562, 570–571
summary overview of, 557, 571
viral, 563–568
  anthropozoonotic potential vs., 563–564
  callitrichid hepatitis as, 566
  filoviruses as, 565
  hepatitis virus as, 565–566
  herpesviruses as, 563–565, 571
  measles as, 563, 571
  paramyxoviruses as, 563
  poxviruses as, 568
  retroviral diseases as, 566–568
  simian retrovirus as, 567, 571
  SIV as, 567, 571
  spumavirus as, 568
  STLV as, 566–567, 571
  yellow fever as, 565
of rabbits, **519–531**
  Cheyletiella spp. as, 522
  Coxiella burnetti as, 522
  Cryptosporidium spp. as, 521
  dermatophytosis as, 522–523
  Encephalitozoon cuniculi as, 521
  enterohemorrhagic *Escherichia coli* as, 520–521
  Francisella tularensis as, 520
  introduction to, 519
  Pasteurella spp. as, 521–522
  summary overview of, 527
  Yersinia pestis as, 519–520
of rodents, **519–531**
  Bartonella spp. as, 523
  Francisella tularensis as, 520
  hantaviruses as, 525
  introduction to, 519
  Leptospira spp. as, 523

lymphocytic choriomeningitis virus as, 525–526
monkeypox virus as, 526
Ornithonyssus bacoti as, 526–527
rabies virus as, bites and exposures from, 513
rat-mite vector of, 526–527
Rickettsia akari as, 524
Rickettsia typhi as, 524–525
Salmonella spp. as, 523–524
Streptobacillus moniliformis as, 524
summary overview of, 527
Yersinia pestis as, 519–520
poultry flock and, **477–490**
    bacterial, 479–483
        Chlamydophila psittaci spp. as, 481–482
        Erysipelothrix rhusiopathiae as, 481
        food-borne, 480
        Mycobacterium avium subspecies *avium* as, 482–483
        Salmonella spp. as, 479–480
    fungal, 486
    parasitic, 486–487
    prevalence of, 477
    prevention recommendations for, 477–479
    summary overview of, 477, 487
    viral, 483–486
        arthropod-borne, 485–486
        avian influenza as, 483–484
        clinical signs of, 483–485
        Newcastle disease as, 484–485
prevention of. See *Prevention of zoonoses.*
rabies as, **507–518**. See also *Rabies virus.*
reportable to CDC, 477
transmission vectors for. See *Vectors.*
wildlife species as reservoir for, 421–423, 491, 500, 552

Printed and bound by CPI Group (UK) Ltd, Croydon, CR0 4YY

03/10/2024

01040448-0015